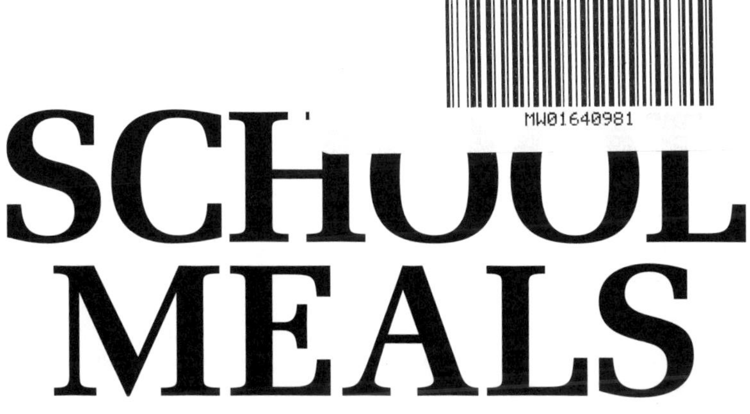

Building Blocks for Healthy Children

Committee on Nutrition Standards for National School Lunch and Breakfast Programs

Food and Nutrition Board

Virginia A. Stallings, Carol West Suitor, and Christine L. Taylor, *Editors*

INSTITUTE OF MEDICINE
OF THE NATIONAL ACADEMIES

THE NATIONAL ACADEMIES PRESS
Washington, D.C.
www.nap.edu

THE NATIONAL ACADEMIES PRESS 500 Fifth Street, N.W. Washington, DC 20001

NOTICE: The project that is the subject of this report was approved by the Governing Board of the National Research Council, whose members are drawn from the councils of the National Academy of Sciences, the National Academy of Engineering, and the Institute of Medicine. The members of the committee responsible for the report were chosen for their special competences and with regard for appropriate balance.

This study was supported by Contract No. AG-3198-C-08-0001 between the National Academy of Sciences and the U.S. Department of Agriculture. Any opinions, findings, conclusions, or recommendations expressed in this publication are those of the author(s) and do not necessarily reflect the view of the organizations or agencies that provided support for this project.

Library of Congress Cataloging-in-Publication Data

Institute of Medicine (U.S.). Committee on Nutrition Standards for National School Lunch and Breakfast Programs.
School meals : building blocks for healthy children / Committee on Nutrition Standards for National School Lunch and Breakfast Programs, Food and Nutrition Board ; Virginia A. Stallings, Carol West Suitor, and Christine L. Taylor, editors.
p. cm.
Includes bibliographical references.
ISBN 978-0-309-14436-0 (pbk.)
1. School children—Food—United States. 2. School children—Nutrition—Government policy—United States. I. Stallings, Virginia A. II. Suitor, Carol West. III. Taylor, Christine Lewis. IV. Title.
[DNLM: 1. Food Services—standards—United States. 2. Nutrition Policy—United States. 3. Adolescent—United States. 4. Child—United States. 5. Schools—United States. WA 350 I59s 2009]
LB3479.U6I67 2009
371.7'16—dc22
2009049798

Additional copies of this report are available from the National Academies Press, 500 Fifth Street, N.W., Lockbox 285, Washington, DC 20055; (800) 624-6242 or (202) 334-3313 (in the Washington metropolitan area); Internet, http://www.nap.edu.

For more information about the Institute of Medicine, visit the IOM home page at: **www.iom.edu**.

Copyright 2010 by the National Academy of Sciences. All rights reserved.

Printed in the United States of America

The serpent has been a symbol of long life, healing, and knowledge among almost all cultures and religions since the beginning of recorded history. The serpent adopted as a logotype by the Institute of Medicine is a relief carving from ancient Greece, now held by the Staatliche Museen in Berlin.

Suggested citation: IOM (Institute of Medicine). 2010. *School Meals: Building Blocks for Healthy Children.* Washington, DC: The National Academies Press.

*"Knowing is not enough; we must apply.
Willing is not enough; we must do."*

—Goethe

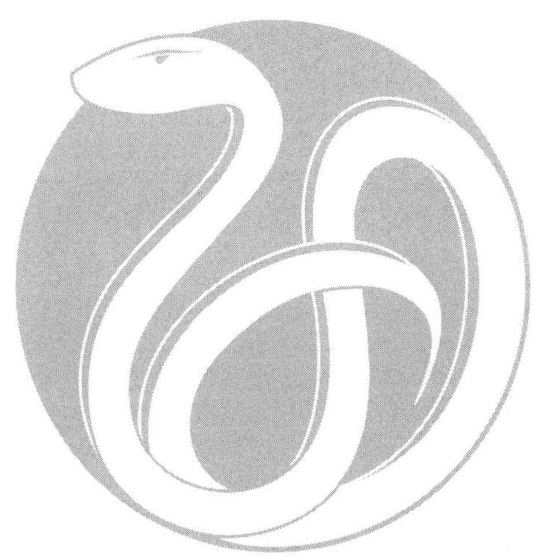

INSTITUTE OF MEDICINE

OF THE NATIONAL ACADEMIES

Advising the Nation. Improving Health.

THE NATIONAL ACADEMIES

Advisers to the Nation on Science, Engineering, and Medicine

The **National Academy of Sciences** is a private, nonprofit, self-perpetuating society of distinguished scholars engaged in scientific and engineering research, dedicated to the furtherance of science and technology and to their use for the general welfare. Upon the authority of the charter granted to it by the Congress in 1863, the Academy has a mandate that requires it to advise the federal government on scientific and technical matters. Dr. Ralph J. Cicerone is president of the National Academy of Sciences.

The **National Academy of Engineering** was established in 1964, under the charter of the National Academy of Sciences, as a parallel organization of outstanding engineers. It is autonomous in its administration and in the selection of its members, sharing with the National Academy of Sciences the responsibility for advising the federal government. The National Academy of Engineering also sponsors engineering programs aimed at meeting national needs, encourages education and research, and recognizes the superior achievements of engineers. Dr. Charles M. Vest is president of the National Academy of Engineering.

The **Institute of Medicine** was established in 1970 by the National Academy of Sciences to secure the services of eminent members of appropriate professions in the examination of policy matters pertaining to the health of the public. The Institute acts under the responsibility given to the National Academy of Sciences by its congressional charter to be an adviser to the federal government and, upon its own initiative, to identify issues of medical care, research, and education. Dr. Harvey V. Fineberg is president of the Institute of Medicine.

The **National Research Council** was organized by the National Academy of Sciences in 1916 to associate the broad community of science and technology with the Academy's purposes of furthering knowledge and advising the federal government. Functioning in accordance with general policies determined by the Academy, the Council has become the principal operating agency of both the National Academy of Sciences and the National Academy of Engineering in providing services to the government, the public, and the scientific and engineering communities. The Council is administered jointly by both Academies and the Institute of Medicine. Dr. Ralph J. Cicerone and Dr. Charles M. Vest are chair and vice chair, respectively, of the National Research Council.

www.national-academies.org

COMMITTEE ON NUTRITION STANDARDS FOR NATIONAL SCHOOL LUNCH AND BREAKFAST PROGRAMS

VIRGINIA A. STALLINGS (*Chair*), The Children's Hospital of Philadelphia, University of Pennsylvania
KAREN WEBER CULLEN, Children's Nutrition Research Center, Baylor College of Medicine, TX
ROSEMARY DEDERICHS, Minneapolis Public Schools, Special School District No. 1, MN
MARY KAY FOX, Mathematica Policy Research, Inc., Cambridge, MA
LISA HARNACK, Division of Epidemiology and Community Health, University of Minnesota, MN
GAIL G. HARRISON, School of Public Health, Center for Health Policy Research, University of California, Los Angeles
MARY ARLINDA HILL, Jackson Public Schools, MS
HELEN H. JENSEN, Department of Economics, Iowa State University, Ames
RONALD E. KLEINMAN, Massachusetts General Hospital for Children, Harvard Medical School, Boston, MA
GEORGE P. McCABE, College of Science, Purdue University, West Lafayette, IN
SUZANNE P. MURPHY, Cancer Research Center of Hawaii, University of Hawaii, Honolulu
ANGELA M. ODOMS-YOUNG, Department of Kinesiology and Nutrition, University of Illinois at Chicago, IL
YEONHWA PARK, Department of Food Science, University of Massachusetts, Amherst
MARY JO TUCKWELL, inTEAM Associates, Ashland, WI

Study Staff

CHRISTINE TAYLOR, Study Director
SHEILA MOATS, Associate Program Officer
JULIA HOGLUND, Research Associate
HEATHER BREINER, Program Associate
CAROL WEST SUITOR, Consultant Subject Matter Expert and Writer
ANTON BANDY, Financial Officer
GERALDINE KENNEDO, Administrative Assistant, Food and Nutrition Board
LINDA D. MEYERS, Director, Food and Nutrition Board

Reviewers

This report has been reviewed in draft form by individuals chosen for their diverse perspectives and technical expertise, in accordance with procedures approved by the National Research Council's (NRC's) Report Review Committee. The purpose of this independent review is to provide candid and critical comments that will assist the institution in making its published report as sound as possible and to ensure that the report meets institutional standards for objectivity, evidence, and responsiveness to the study charge. The review comments and draft manuscript remain confidential to protect the integrity of the deliberative process. We wish to thank the following individuals for their review of this report:

Cheryl A. M. Anderson, Department of Epidemiology, The Johns Hopkins Bloomberg School of Public Health, Baltimore, MD
Janet Currie, Economics Department, Columbia University, New York, NY
Barbara L. Devaney, Human Services Research, Research Division, Mathematica Policy Research, Inc., Boston, MA
Deanna M. Hoelscher, School of Public Health, University of Texas Health Sciences Center at Houston
Eileen T. Kennedy, Friedman School of Nutrition Sciences and Policy, Tufts University, Boston, MA
Daryl Lund, Cottage Grove, WI
Penny McConnell, Food and Nutrition Services, Fairfax County Public Schools, Vienna, VA
Barry Sackin, B. Sackin & Associates, L.L.C., Murrieta, CA

Sandra Schlicker, Wellness and Nutrition Services, Office of the State Superintendent of Education, Government of the District of Columbia, Washington, DC
Frances H. Seligson, Independent Consultant, Hershey, PA
Patricia Wahl, University of Washington School of Public Health and Community Medicine, Seattle
Walter C. Willett, Department of Nutrition, Harvard School of Public Health, Boston, MA

Although the reviewers listed above have provided many constructive comments and suggestions, they were not asked to endorse the conclusions or recommendations nor did they see the final draft of the report before its release. The review of this report was overseen by **Elaine L. Larson**, School of Nursing, Columbia University, and **Joanna T. Dwyer**, Tufts University School of Medicine & Friedman School of Nutrition Science & Policy, Frances Stern Nutrition Center, Tufts-New England Medical Centers. Appointed by the NRC and Institute of Medicine, they were responsible for making certain that an independent examination of this report was carried out in accordance with institutional procedures and that all review comments were carefully considered. Responsibility for the final content of this report rests entirely with the authoring committee and the institution.

Preface

My small southern town memories of food at school are many, starting with cafeteria lunch provided after we presented our green tokens and without discussion of choices or options except for the big decision of chocolate or plain milk. Everyone had a lunch token, so no one knew that there was a free or reduced-price lunch and no one went home or off campus for lunch unless you lived in the neighborhood. Bigger or maybe hungrier students got larger portions. A few students brought lunch in cool lunch boxes, and we envied what was assumed to be a better lunch. There were no vending machines until high school, and then the machine foods and beverages were few, and most students did not come to school with money or plans to purchase foods other than school lunch. We did not want to spend our allowance on food.

This was a time when childhood nutrition issues were iron deficiency and undernutrition, when few were concerned about fat, sugar, or sodium in childhood diets, and when most meals were consumed at home with family members or at school. I now know that some children were hungry and the school lunch, and later school breakfast, was an important source of food. Interestingly, the key stakeholders have not changed—the children, families, school administrators, teachers, nurses, coaches, food service team, and food industry. The local and state school authorities implement federal policy and make many food and health decisions at their levels. In the background, nutritionists, health-care providers, and other child advocates influence both policy and implementation. We now clearly recognize the importance of food and nutrient intake on child health and on lifelong adult health. All stakeholders are concerned about diet quality and quantity, emerging food and health habits, and maintaining a healthy pattern of childhood growth. Today overweight children outnumber undernourished children, and childhood obesity is often referred to as an epidemic in both the medical and community settings. Nonetheless, normal or overweight status does not guarantee food security and a healthful diet for many children. Our inexpensive, abundant food supply and innovative food industry provide highly palatable foods and beverages for children. School foods and beverages, once almost limited mainly to school lunch, now often include many choices in addition to the meals offered by federally supported school breakfast and lunch programs. The calories and nutrients consumed at school and school-related activities are an important component of dietary intake of all school-age children.

It is within this scientific and social environment that our committee established criteria for nutrient targets and meal standards and made recommendations to revise the nutrition- and food-related standards and requirements for the National School Lunch Program and the School Breakfast Program. The recommended standards for menu planning lay out a school meal approach that results in the wide array of nutrients that children need and that reflect the *Dietary Guidelines for Americans*.

Our committee is a dedicated group of remarkable people from diverse backgrounds and experiences. We quickly recognized that this was not an easy task. Over nearly 2 years, we learned and debated together, and developed this set of recommendations for nutrition and food standards for schools meals. We recognized that the standards will be effective only to the extent that standards are implemented effectively and thus made recommendations related to technical support, developing foods that are reduced in sodium content, and taking measures to help schools incorporate more products that are rich in whole grains.

The goal is for schools to employ their unique, long-term relationship with children and their families to support child health and provide a healthful school eating environment. This will require attention to many factors that go beyond the federally supported school meal programs: competitive foods (foods and beverages offered other than the meals provided under the National School Lunch and Breakfast programs), time and duration of meal periods, activity level of children, and evaluation and research that address interactions of such factors with the success of the school meal programs.

The involvement of students, parents, schools, and the food industry is important to the success of implementing the recommended revisions. Support from state and federal agencies and from professional organizations and child advocacy groups will help to promote the acceptance of the recommended meals. Finally, the level of federal reimbursement for school meals needs to be sufficient to cover the cost of improvements in the meals such as increased amounts of fruits and vegetables and the substitution of whole grain-rich foods for some of the refined grains.

Sincere appreciation is extended to the many individuals and groups who were instrumental in the development of this report. First and foremost, many thanks are due to the committee members, who volunteered countless hours to the research, deliberations, and preparation of the report. Their dedication to this project was outstanding and is the basis of our success.

Many individuals volunteered significant time and effort to address and educate our committee members during our two public workshops on July 8, 2008, and January 28, 2009. Workshop speakers included: Tom Baranowski, Kimberly Barnes-O'Connor, Jessica Donze Black, Helene Clark, Adalia Espinosa, Joanne F. Guthrie, Jeanne Harris, Geraldine Henchy, Fred Higgens, Jay Hirschman, Lynn Hoggard, Sue E. Holbert, Leonard Marquart, Cathie McCullough, Celeste Peggs, Matt Sharp, Ted Spitzer, Kimberly Stizel, Katie Wilson, and Margo Wootan.

In addition representatives from many entities provided oral testimony to the committee during the public workshops that were held on July 8, 2009, and January 28, 2009. They represented the Action for Healthy Kids, Alliance for a Healthier Generation, American Academy of Pediatrics, American Dietetic Association, Apple Processors Association, ARMARK Education, Baylor College of Medicine, Food Research and Action Center, California Food Policy Advocates, Charterwells School Dining Services, Economic Research Service, Food Distribution Program and Food and Nutrition Service of United States Department of Agriculture, General Mills, Grocery Manufacturers Association, International Dairy Foods Association, Local Matters, National Alliance for Nutrition and Activity, National Dairy Council, National Pork Board, Nemours Division of Health and Prevention Services, School Nutrition Association, Soyfoods Association of North America, Sunkist Taylor LLC, United Egg Producers, United Fresh Produce Association, University of Minnesota, U.S. Apple Association, and Wellness in American Schools.

It is apparent that many organizations and individuals from a variety of school and scientific backgrounds provided timely and essential support for this project. Yet we would have never succeeded without the extensive contributions of Carol West Suitor, ScD, as Consultant Subject Matter Expert and Writer to the project. Furthermore, it is important to recognize the efforts, skills, and grace that were provided in large measure by Christine L. Taylor, PhD, RD, Study Director for this project; Sheila Moats, BS, Associate Program Officer; Julia Hoglund, MPH, Research Associate; Heather Breiner, BS, Program Associate; and Linda Meyers, PhD, Director, Food and Nutrition Board. I also want to thank Todd Campbell from Iowa State University for developing the software used by the committee to analyze menus for cost and nutrient analyses, and Mathematica Policy Research, Inc. for providing data analyses. Last, as chair, I express my sincere appreciation to each member of this committee for their extraordinary commitment to the project and the wonderful opportunity to work with them on this important task for the nutrition and school communities and for the schoolchildren whose health and future we were asked to consider.

Virginia A. Stallings, *Chair*
Committee on Nutrition Standards for National
School Lunch and Breakfast Programs

Contents

APPENDIXES*

*Appendixes C through Q are not printed in this book, but can be found on the CD at the back of the book or online at http://www.nap.edu.

Summary

Ensuring that the foods[1] provided to children in schools are consistent with current dietary recommendations is an important national focus. The National School Lunch Program (NSLP) and the School Breakfast Program (SBP) hold the potential to provide nearly all the nation's schoolchildren with access to nutritious, low-cost meals to support their growth, development, and health. The NSLP alone is available in 99 percent of U.S. public schools and in 83 percent of private and public schools. In fiscal year 2007, the participating schools served about 5.1 billion lunches at a federal cost of approximately $8.7 billion. If a school participates in one or both of the school meal programs, any child who attends the school may have access to the school meal.

Various laws and regulations govern the operation of the school meal programs. In 1995, new Nutrition Standards and Meal Requirements were put in place to ensure that the meals offered will be of high nutritional quality. The eight recommendations in this report update those Nutrition Standards and Meal Requirements, shift the focus toward meeting recommendations in *Dietary Guidelines for Americans*, emphasize the need for effective implementation, and identify key research topics.

Numerous school-based factors, such as other foods offered and nutrition education efforts, ultimately have an impact on the foods that children eat at school. Many are not related to Nutrition Standards and Meal Requirements and, therefore, are beyond the scope of this report. Nonetheless, these standards and requirements provide the starting point for the complex

[1]The word *foods* is meant to encompass both foods and beverages.

journey to improving the diets of a vulnerable and important population group, our children.

THE TASK

The U.S. Department of Agriculture (USDA) requested that the Institute of Medicine (IOM) provide recommendations to revise the nutrition- and food-related standards and requirements for the NSLP and the SBP. This request relates to the congressional requirement that USDA issue new guidance and regulations for the Nutrition Standards and Meal Requirements of the school meal programs.

In particular, the committee was asked to review and assess the food and nutritional needs of school-aged children in the United States using the 2005 *Dietary Guidelines for Americans* and the IOM's Dietary Reference Intakes (DRIs) and to use that review as a basis for recommended revisions to the NSLP and SBP Nutrition Standards and Meal Requirements. The goal was the development of a set of well-conceived, practical, and economical recommendations for standards that reflect current nutritional science, increase the availability of key food groups as appropriate, and allow these two meal programs to better meet the nutritional needs of children, foster healthy eating habits, and safeguard children's health. Both a Phase I report and a final report were to be prepared.

Figure S-1 depicts the current relationships among major elements of the task, focusing on the Nutrition Standards and Meal Requirements. The figure uses a number of the terms that are specific to school meal programs and depicts the two existing approaches to menu planning, one that relies on a food-based approach and one that relies on a nutrient-based approach.

In the course of its work, the committee made recommendations that require a change in terminology and a revised approach to menu planning that leads to a less complex set of elements for the planning of school meals (see Figure S-2, and compare it with Figure S-1). In particular, the committee provides recommendations for (1) Nutrient Targets rather than Nutrition Standards and (2) only one method of menu planning rather than several. It uses the phrase *as selected by the student* rather than *as served* to provide clarity. The recommended Nutrient Targets provide the foundation for setting revised Meal Requirements. The recommended Meal Requirements encompass meal patterns and other specifications for menu planning (the standards for menu planning) and specifications for the number and types of food that the student must select for a reimbursable meal (the standards for meals *as selected* by the student).

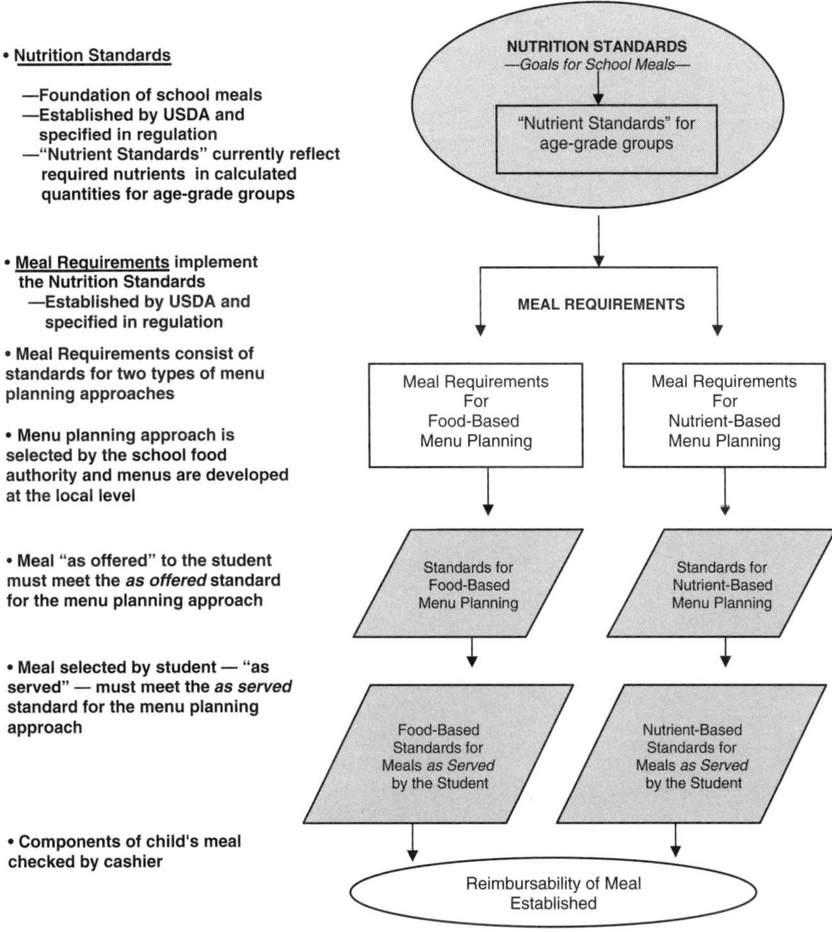

FIGURE S-1 Relationships among *current* Nutrition Standards, Meal Requirements, and eligibility for federal reimbursement.

THE APPROACH

During Phase I of the project, the committee developed four criteria to guide the development and testing of its recommendations, proposed a process for addressing its tasks, and prepared the Phase I report for public comment. The final version of the criteria appears in Box S-1.

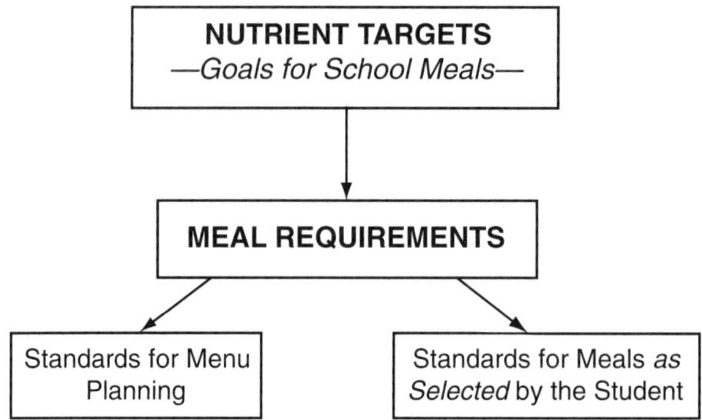

FIGURE S-2 Depiction of the *recommended* elements in the path to nutritious school meals. In this figure and throughout the remainder of the report, the committee uses the term *as selected by the student* (or simply *as selected*) rather than *as served* to apply to standards for reimbursable meals.

BOX S-1
Criteria for the Nutrient Targets and Meal Requirements for the National School Lunch Program and the School Breakfast Program

Criterion 1. The Nutrient Targets and Meal Requirements will be consistent with current dietary guidance and nutrition recommendations to promote health—as exemplified by the *Dietary Guidelines for Americans* and the Dietary Reference Intakes—with the ultimate goals of improving children's diets by reducing the prevalence of inadequate and excessive intakes of food, nutrients, and calories.

Criterion 2. The Nutrient Targets and Meal Requirements will be considered on the basis of age-grade groups that are consistent with the current age-gender categories used for specifying reference values and with widely used school grade configurations.

Criterion 3. The Nutrient Targets and Meal Requirements will result in the simplification of the menu planning and monitoring processes, and they will be compatible with the development of menus that are practical to prepare and serve and that offer nutritious foods and beverages that appeal to students of diverse cultural backgrounds.

Criterion 4. The Nutrient Targets and Meal Requirements will be sensitive to program costs and school administrative concerns.

During this second phase of the work, the approach used to develop the recommended Nutrient Targets and Meal Requirements involved

- setting age-grade groups,
- conducting a new review of schoolchildren's dietary intakes using data from the third School Nutrition Dietary Assessment study (SNDA-III),
- testing methods of setting the Nutrient Targets,
- using preliminary targets in developing Meal Requirements, and
- checking possible requirements against the four criteria.

Extensive analyses provided the foundation for the recommended Nutrient Targets and Meal Requirements. The process of developing the recommendations was iterative. For example, initial proposals for the Meal Requirements were tested to determine how well they aligned with the committee's criteria, and the results were used to modify the proposals to achieve a better fit. The final products—the recommended Nutrient Targets and Meal Requirements—are described in detail in the report.

NUTRIENT TARGETS

Currently, Nutrition Standards provide the basis for nutrient-based menu planning and the monitoring of meal quality every 5 years, but the committee decided that this approach does not necessarily lead to meals that are consistent with the *Dietary Guidelines*. Furthermore, nutrient-based menu planning is unnecessarily complex if a broad array of nutrients is to be considered. Therefore, the committee developed the concept of Nutrient Targets to replace Nutrition Standards. The Nutrient Targets would provide the scientific basis of the standards for menu planning, but they would be only one of the elements considered when developing these standards.

Recommended Nutrient Targets

Recommendation 1. The Food and Nutrition Service of USDA should adopt the Nutrient Targets as the scientific basis for setting standards for menu planning for school meals but should not adopt a nutrient-based standard for school meal planning and monitoring.

To ensure that all nutrient recommendations were considered, the committee set targets for 24 nutrients and other dietary components. Because the Nutrient Targets are intended for developing standards for menu planning that are consistent with the DRIs and not for planning actual menus, it was desirable to set Nutrient Targets for most nutrients with a DRI. Key aspects of the Nutrient Targets appear below.

Calories

In contrast to the current standard for calories, which specifies only a minimum calorie level, both minimum and maximum calorie levels for breakfast and lunch are recommended for each age group (5–10 years, kindergarten through grade 5; 11–13 years, grades 6 through 8; and 14–18 years, grades 9 through 12). The recommendations are based on reference growth chart data for healthy weights and heights, objective data on physical activity, and data on how calories are distributed among meals and snacks consumed by schoolchildren. Maximum calorie levels are introduced in part because of concern about the high prevalence of childhood overweight and obesity in the United States. The recommended calorie levels are either lower or comparable to the existing *minimum* calorie standard. The meals offer adequate amounts of nutrients, and the level of calories is appropriate for the level of physical activity of most children.

Fats and Cholesterol

One change was made in setting the targets for fats and cholesterol: the recommended upper limit for total fat was *increased* from 30 to 35 percent of the calories. This aligns the target with *Dietary Guidelines*. Although the goal is to eliminate *trans* fat from school meals, it was not possible to set a specific Nutrient Target for this fat. However, the standards for menu planning set zero grams of *trans* fat as the amount declared on the label of foods used in school meals. The target for saturated fat, which is less than 10 percent of calories, is unchanged.

Protein, Vitamins, and Minerals

To set recommended Nutrient Targets for protein and selected vitamins and minerals, the committee used an adaptation of the Target Median Intake (TMI) method. This method, recommended by the IOM, is designed to identify the change in intake of each nutrient that would be likely to reduce the predicted prevalence of inadequacy to a specific level. Because school meals are consumed by subgroups of children with differing calorie and nutrient needs within an age-grade group, the committee considered the ratio of nutrient needs (based on the Estimated Average Requirement or Adequate Intake) relative to the calorie requirements (based on the Estimated Energy Requirement) for each subgroup within a school meals age-

BOX S-2
Key Aspects of Recommended Nutrient Targets

- Nutrient Targets are recommended for use in the development of the standards for menu planning, not for menu planning or for monitoring of the nutritional quality of the meals.
- Recommended targets cover both minimum and maximum calorie levels.
- The number of specifications increased from 8 requirements to 24 targets for nutrients and other dietary components.

grade group. For example, because females ages 14–18 years have higher nutrient requirements relative to their calorie needs than do males of the same age, the School Meal-TMIs for this age group were set based on the needs of the females.

This approach results in Nutrient Targets that will meet the needs of more children than would past approaches based on Recommended Dietary Allowances. Even though the targets are relatively high, analyses of projected intakes indicate a low prevalence of intakes that exceed the Tolerable Upper Intake Level for most nutrients. Furthermore, analyses showed that almost all the Nutrient Targets would be met if MyPyramid food patterns, which correspond to the *Dietary Guidelines for Americans*, are used as the basis of standards for menu planning (see next section).

For protein, vitamins, and minerals at lunch, the recommended Nutrient Targets are set at 32 percent of the School Meal-TMI. At breakfast, they are set at 21.5 percent of the School Meal-TMI. (For sodium, the target is the corresponding percentage of the Tolerable Upper Intake Level.) Although a Nutrient Target has not been set for vitamin D, the standards for menu planning described below ensure that children are offered at least 8 fluid ounces of milk at each meal, which provides one-half of the Adequate Intake for vitamin D at each meal.

Key aspects of the recommended Nutrient Targets appear in Box S-2.

RECOMMENDED MEAL REQUIREMENTS

The Meal Requirements encompass two types of standards: (1) standards for menu planning and (2) standards for meals *as selected* by the student.

Standards for Menu Planning

Recommendation 2. To align school meals with the *Dietary Guidelines for Americans* and improve the healthfulness of school meals, the Food and Nutrition Service should adopt standards for menu planning that increase the amounts of fruits, vegetables, and whole grains; increase the focus on reducing the amounts of saturated fat and sodium provided; and set a minimum and maximum level of calories—as presented in Table S-1.

The recommendation is for a *single* approach to menu planning that is largely food based but that also includes specifications for minimum and maximum calorie levels, maximum saturated fat content, and maximum sodium content. Without those specifications, there would be no practical way to achieve alignment with *Dietary Guidelines*.

The recommended standards for planning menus for school breakfasts (see Table S-2) cover the weekly amounts of food from five of the food groups and subgroups listed under "Meal Pattern" in the table (including both whole grain-rich and refined grains) and specifications expressed as a 5-day average for three dietary components: calories, saturated fat, and sodium. The recommended standards for school lunches cover the weekly amounts of food from all 10 food groups and subgroups listed under "Meal Pattern" and specifications for the same three dietary components. As designed, these standards lead to menus that meet or are very close to the Nutrient Targets for all but four or five nutrients (depending on the meal and the age-grade group) when the nutrient content is averaged over a 5-day school week. The exceptions were expected, as explained in Chapter 9 of the report.

Standards for Meals *as Selected* by the Student

Recommendation 3. To achieve a reasonable balance between the goals of reducing waste and preserving the nutritional integrity of school meals, the Food and Nutrition Service, in conjunction with state and local educational agencies and students, should weigh the strengths and limitations of the committee's two options (see Table S-2) when setting standards for the meals *as selected* by the student.

Noting that Congress has specified the various types of stakeholders that are to be involved in the initial design phase for administrative procedures for meals *as served*, the committee developed two options for the standards for meals *as selected* by the student and identified strengths and limitations of each. The options differ in the number of food items that may be declined, but they both include a new requirement related to the

TABLE S-1 Recommended *as Offered* Meal Standards

	Breakfast			Lunch		
	Grades K–5	Grades 6–8	Grades 9–12	Grades K–5	Grades 6–8	Grades 9–12
Meal Pattern	Amount of Foods[a] Per Week					
Fruits (cups)[b]	5	5	5	2.5	2.5	5
Vegetables (cups)[b]	0	0	0	3.75	3.75	5
Dark green	0	0	0	0.5[c]	0.5[c]	0.5[c]
Orange	0	0	0	0.5[c]	0.5[c]	0.5[c]
Legumes	0	0	0	0.5[c]	0.5[c]	0.5[c]
Starchy	0	0	0	1	1	1
Other	0	0	0	1.25[c]	1.25[c]	2.5[c]
Grains, at least half of which must be whole grain-rich[d] (oz eq)	7–10	8–10	9–10	9–10	9–10	12–13
Meats, beans, cheese, yogurt (oz eq)	5	5	7–10	8–10	9–10	10–12
Fat-free milk (plain or flavored) or low-fat milk (1% milk fat or less) (cups)	5	5	5	5	5	5
Other Specifications	Other Specifications: Daily Amount Based on the Average for a 5-Day Week					
Min-max calories (kcal)[e,f]	350–500	400–550	450–600	550–650	600–700	750–850
Saturated fat (% of total calories)[g]	< 10	< 10	< 10	< 10	< 10	< 10
Sodium (mg)	[≤ 430]	[≤ 470]	[≤ 500]	[≤ 640]	[≤ 710]	[≤ 740]
	Sodium targets are to be reached by the year 2020.[h]					
trans fat	Nutrition label must specify zero grams of *trans* fat per serving.[i]					

NOTES: K = kindergarten; kcal = calories; max = maximum; mg = milligrams; min = minimum; oz eq = ounce equivalent. Although the recommended weekly meal intake patterns do not specify amounts of unsaturated oils, their use is to be encouraged within calorie limits.

[a]Food items included in each group and subgroup and amount equivalents. Appendix Table H-1 gives a listing of foods by food group and subgroup. Minimum daily requirements apply: 1/5 of the weekly requirement for fruits, total vegetables, and milk and at least 1oz equivalent each of grains and meat or meat alternate (2 oz of each for grades 9–12 lunch).

[b]One cup of fruits and vegetables usually provides two servings; ¼ cup of dried fruit counts as ½ cup of fruit; 1 cup of leafy greens counts as ½ cup of vegetables. No more than half of the fruit offerings may be in the form of juice.

[c]Larger amounts of these vegetables may be served.

[d]Based on at least half of the grain content as whole grain. Aiming for a higher proportion of whole grain-rich foods is encouraged. See Box 7-1 for Temporary Criterion for Whole-Grain Rich Foods. Also note that in Chapter 10 the committee recommends that the Food Buying Guide serving sizes be updated to be consistent with MyPyramid Equivalent serving sizes.

[e]The average daily amount for a 5-day school week is not to be less than the minimum or exceed the maximum.

[f]Discretionary sources of calories (for example, solid fats and added sugars) may be added to the meal pattern if within the specifications for calories, saturated fat, *trans* fat, and sodium.

[g]The average daily amount for a 5-day school week is not to exceed the maximum.

[h]To ensure that action is taken to reduce the sodium content of school meals over the 10-year period in a manner that maintains student participation rates, the committee suggests the setting of intermediate targets for each 2-year interval. (See the section "Achieving Long-Term Goals" in Chapter 10.)

[i]Because the nutrition facts panel is not required for foods with Child Nutrition labeling, the committee suggests that only products with 0 grams of *trans* fat per serving be eligible for consideration for such labeling.

TABLE S-2 Options for Standards for Meals *as Selected* by the Student under the *Offer Versus Serve* Provision of P.L. 94-105[a]

	Number of Items the Student May Decline and Required Items	
	Breakfast	Lunch
1. Preferred	One item[b] may be declined, must take at least one fruit or juice	Two items may be declined, must take at least one fruit or vegetable
2. Alternative	Two items may be declined, must take at least one fruit or juice	Three items may be declined, must take at least one fruit or vegetable

NOTE: Options are provided for consideration by the U.S. Department of Agriculture, working cooperatively with state educational agencies and with participation by local educational agencies and student to develop new regulations.

[a]Under current traditional food-based menu planning standards, high school students are required to take 3 out of 4 (or 5) food items at breakfast and 3 out of 5 food items at lunch. *Offer versus serve* is optional for elementary and middle schools.

[b]A specific food offered in the specified portion sizes that will meet the recommended *as offered* Meal Standards.

selection of a fruit or vegetable. A rule that allows more options to decline foods clearly could reduce waste, but it would increase the chance that the nutritional integrity of the children's meals would not be maintained, and vice versa. Foods need to be appealing to students to encourage selection and consumption.

Summary of Changes in the Meal Requirements

Major changes in the Meal Requirements are summarized in Box S-3.

RECOMMENDATIONS FOR IMPLEMENTATION AND MONITORING

The Meal Requirements will be beneficial only to the extent that program participation is maintained or increased and the participants' food consumption improves. The effectiveness of revised Meal Requirements will be determined in a large part by the manner in which they are implemented. Strategies that can be used to promote change include engaging the school community; involving students, parents, and the community; providing nutrition education; training and mentoring of food service workers; and providing technical assistance. An essential element of the implementation processes will be industry involvement to develop appealing foods that are lower in sodium and saturated fat and that have a higher ratio of whole grain to refined grain. Effective monitoring can lead to improvements in implementation efforts.

BOX S-3
Major Recommended Changes in the Meal Requirements

Meal Planning Approaches

- The recommended approach to meal planning is food-based with the additions of quantitative specifications for minimum and maximum calorie levels, maximum saturated fat content, and maximum sodium content.
- Only one approach to menu planning is recommended.
- Computer analysis of nutrient content could be used to assist in planning menus that meet the recommended standards for menu planning but would not be needed to analyze the vitamin and mineral content of meals.

Standards for Menu Planning

- The standards for all age-grade groups include more food groups and introduce food subgroups. More fruit is specified. Fruits and vegetables are not interchangeable.
- Specifications for types of food to be included are more precise.
  - Over a 5-day school week,
    - The average daily calorie content of the meal offerings must be within the specified minimum and maximum levels and the average saturated fat content must be less than 10 percent of calories.
    - Vegetable offerings at lunch must include at least one-half cup equivalent of each of the following: dark green vegetables, bright orange vegetables, and legumes.
    - No more than half of the fruit offerings may be in the form of juice.
    - At least half of the bread/grain offerings must meet the criterion for a whole grain-rich food (based on at least half of the grain content as whole grain, see Box 7-1 in Chapter 7).
  - On a daily basis,
    - The milk must be fat-free (plain or flavored) or plain low-fat (1 percent milk fat or less).
    - If purchased commercially, the nutrition labeling or manufacturer's specification must indicate that the product contains zero grams of *trans* fat per serving.
    - The inclusion of unsaturated vegetable oils is encouraged within calorie limits.

Standards for Foods That Are Selected by the Student

- Two options are presented, and the strengths and limitations of each are described in the text. Both options specify that the student must select a fruit at breakfast and either a fruit or vegetable at lunch for the meal to be reimbursable.

Recommendation 4. The Food and Nutrition Service, working together with state agencies, professional organizations, and industry, should provide extensive support to enable food service operators to adapt to the many changes required by revised Meal Requirements. The types of support required include the following:

a. Technical assistance for developing and continuously improving menus, ordering appropriate foods (including the writing of specifications), and controlling costs while maintaining quality.

b. New procedures for monitoring the quality of school meals that (1) focus on meeting relevant *Dietary Guidelines* and (2) provide information for continuous quality improvement and for mentoring food service workers to assist in performance improvement.

It is essential that USDA collaborate with school food service directors to revise related menu planning guidance materials, including the *Food Buying Guide for Child Nutrition Programs*. The committee encourages the simplification of procedures for selecting specific foods in amounts that will meet the standards.

The committee suggests that, at least for the next few years, monitoring guidance be directed toward facilitating the transition to the new Meal Requirements. Such guidance would place an emphasis on examining progress in meeting the standards, especially those related to fruits, vegetables, whole grain-rich foods, calories, saturated fat, and sodium; identifying training needs for school food service operators; and providing needed technical assistance to improve the school meals.

Recommendation 5. USDA should work cooperatively with Health and Human Services, the food industry, professional organizations, state agencies, advocacy groups, and parents to develop strategies and incentives to reduce the sodium content of prepared foods and to increase the availability of whole grain-rich products while maintaining acceptable palatability, cost, and safety.

The specification for sodium merits special attention. The committee recognizes that there are barriers to reducing the sodium content of meals to the recommended levels without having long-term adverse effects on student acceptance and participation, safety, practicality, and cost. For this reason, the committee set the year 2020 as the date to achieve full implementation; and it suggests that intermediate targets be set at 2-year intervals and be periodically re-evaluated to promote stepwise reductions in sodium content over the decade beginning in 2010.

Recommendation 6. The Food and Drug Administration should take action to require labeling for the whole grain content of food products.

The lack of such labeling is a major barrier to menu planners who are striving to achieve at least a one-to-one ratio of whole grains to refined grains, as recommended by *Dietary Guidelines*.

CONSISTENCY OF RECOMMENDATIONS WITH THE COMMITTEE'S CRITERIA

The recommendations for Nutrient Targets and Meal Requirements and for implementing and monitoring them are consistent with the committee's criteria, as summarized below.

Criterion 1. Consistent with Current Dietary Guidance

The Nutrient Targets were based on the Dietary Reference Intakes, using methods recommended for this purpose. The Meal Requirements were designed to come as close as possible to *Dietary Guidelines* and to the Nutrient Targets while still being practical. Sample menus were reviewed to confirm their consistency with *Dietary Guidelines* (see Box S-4) and were analyzed to confirm reasonable consistency with the recommended Nutrient Targets. Chapter 10 addresses strategies to reduce the sodium content and to increase whole grains in school meals to bring them into closer alignment with *Dietary Guidelines.*

Dietary Guidelines emphasize meeting nutrient needs without exceeding energy needs. The ranges for the calorie content of school meals reflect the best judgment of the committee based on current evidence for the energy requirements of schoolchildren. The committee recognizes that there is a wider range of actual requirements, but it set the ranges with the objective of avoiding the provision of excessive calories while ensuring the offering of amounts of vitamins, minerals, and protein that would be appropriate

BOX S-4
Recommended Changes in Standards for Menu Planning Improve Alignment with *Dietary Guidelines for Americans*

- Both a minimum and a maximum calorie level
- More fruit at breakfast, including whole fruit
- A greater amount and variety of vegetables at lunch
- Both fruit and vegetables required on the lunch menu
- More whole grain-rich foods, fewer refined grain foods
- Milk choices limited to fat-free (unflavored or flavored) and plain low-fat (1 percent milk fat or less)
- Increased emphasis on limiting saturated fat
- Encouragement to include unsaturated oils within the calorie limits
- Minimized content of *trans* fat
- Major reduction in sodium content to be achieved fully by the year 2020, with stepwise reductions

for essentially all children in the age-grade group. The high nutrient quality of the meals supports the role that school meals play as a safety net in meeting the nutrient needs of children who may be at risk for inadequate food intake and food insecurity.

Criterion 2. Appropriate Age-Grade Groups

The age-grade groups established by the committee consider the current age-gender categories used in the DRIs to the extent that they are compatible with widely used school grade configurations. The committee made adjustments to account for differences between the Dietary Reference Intake age groupings and school grade configurations—for the kindergarten through grade 5 group in particular. Because differences are small between the standards for meal planning for the elementary and middle school groupings, food service operators may plan identical menus for children in kindergarten through grade 8 if applicable to the local food service operation.

Criterion 3. Simplified Menu Planning and Monitoring and Student Acceptance of School Meals

Simplification of Menu Planning

The committee worked to develop the least complex approach to menu planning that would be consistent with *Dietary Guidelines*. Although the recommended standards for menu planning are not as simple as the current food-based standards, it was essential to introduce new elements to conform to *Dietary Guidelines*. The committee ruled out making recommendations for nutrient-based menu planning because there was not a practical way to do so that would cover the full array of nutrients and also ensure consistency with *Dietary Guidelines*.

High-quality menu planning for school meals is always a complex task, and application of the standards for menu planning will present challenges for many school food service directors. However, meeting the Meal Requirements is only one of many aspects of the process. Chapter 10 addresses a number of approaches that would help menu planners to gradually implement the new standards for menu planning. Recommendation 4a in the previous section emphasizes how important it will be for food service operators to receive technical support and other forms of assistance to implement the new Meal Requirements.

From a broader programmatic perspective, the standards have been simplified (for example, compare Figure S-2 with Figure S-1). Recommendations provide for a single, primarily food-based approach to menu planning and three consistent age-grade groups for breakfast and lunch. They provide the means to meet *Dietary Guidelines* rather than focusing on meeting all the Nutrient Targets. Required food composition data are limited to calories, saturated fat, *trans* fat, and sodium—each of which is readily available on nutrition facts panels or from manufacturers.

Simplification of Monitoring the Nutritional Quality of Meals

Recommendation 4b concerning the monitoring of the quality of school meals does not call for analysis of the broad array of nutrients for which Nutrient Targets were set. Instead, the monitoring process would be designed to help schools improve their menus and food service operation in ways that produce appealing meals that meet the recommended Meal Requirements and control overall costs.

Basis for Practical and Appealing Nutritious Meals

The committee used the meal patterns to develop 4 weeks of practical and appealing nutritious menus for breakfast and lunch for each of the three age-grade groups.

Criterion 4. Sensitive to Costs and Administrative Concerns

Measures to help school food programs meet *Dietary Guidelines* will increase costs and the need for administrative support. Largely because of increases in the recommended amounts of fruits, vegetables, and whole grain-rich foods, menu costs are expected to increase, especially for the school breakfast. By estimating the costs of representative baseline menus and comparing them with those of baseline menus modified by the committee to meet the recommendations, the committee found that the foods costs for breakfast (*as selected* by the student) increased by 18 percent, largely because of the increase in fruit, and those for lunch (*as selected*) increased by 4 percent. These estimates are representative of the expected increase in food costs that are due to the recommended changes in menus, but they should be viewed with some caution, especially because students' food selections under the new Meal Requirements cannot be known in advance. If even higher percentages of students select the maximum amount of fruits and vegetables, the food costs for breakfast and lunch may increase up to 23 percent and 9 percent, respectively. Furthermore, price changes that reflect changes in the market for food products important in the school meal programs (such as dairy and fruits) can have a significant effect on the cost of meals.

The committee recognizes that, at current federal reimbursement levels, most school food authorities will be unable to absorb these increased costs completely, even with better management. Implementation of the recommended Meal Requirements likely will require some combination of higher federal meal reimbursement, a source of capital investment to cover costs of equipment, and additional money to train operators to prepare more food from basic ingredients.

Other school administrative concerns relate to potential changes in student participation, the menu planning process, purchasing, preparation and meal service, routine monitoring, the staffing pattern, staff training, equipment, and kitchen and storeroom space. The committee considered all these elements in the development of the Meal Requirements. With the adoption of appropriate implementation strategies, the changes in student participation rates are expected to be temporary and relatively small and, thus, to have limited administrative impact. The committee recognizes that some administrative changes will be necessary. For a smooth transition, technical assistance must cover analysis of and strategies for the most effective approaches to implementing menu changes.

RECOMMENDATIONS FOR EVALUATION AND RESEARCH

The committee considered needs for the overall evaluation of the Nutrient Targets and Meal Requirements and for related research. Key recommendations follow:

Recommendation 7. Relevant agencies in USDA and other federal departments should provide support for the conduct of studies to evaluate the revised Meal Requirements for the School Breakfast Program and the National School Lunch Program.

a. USDA should continue funding for periodic School Nutrition Dietary Assessment studies, with the intermittent addition of a cost component.

b. USDA should take the lead in providing funding to conduct well-designed short-term studies in varied school settings to better understand how the new Meal Requirements change children's total and school meal dietary intakes, student participation, food service operations, and cost.

Recommendation 8. The committee recommends that agencies of USDA, of other federal departments, and relevant foundations fund research studies on topics related to the implementation of the new Meal Requirements, children's acceptance of and participation in school meals, and children's health—especially the following:

a. Effects of the recommended range of calorie levels on the adequacy of energy intakes for individual children within each of the age-grade categories.

b. Impacts of various approaches to reducing the sodium content of school meals and student acceptance of reduced-sodium foods.

c. Impacts of various approaches to increase the acceptance of whole grain-rich products.

d. Fruit and vegetable options and preparation methods that will increase consumption and decrease waste.

e. Effects on cost, waste, and food and nutrient intakes of various options to govern the number and types of foods students must accept for a reimbursable meal under the *offer versus serve* provision of the law.

f. Targeted approaches to decreasing the prevalence of nutrient inadequacy that do not require increasing the intakes of all children.

g. Changes in child health as a result of the new standards.

CLOSING REMARKS

The recommendations for Nutrient Targets and Meal Requirements lay the foundation for healthy school meals that are consistent with current dietary recommendations. The ultimate effect of improvements in program regulations that are based on these recommendations will depend on the effectiveness of a broad array of implementation strategies. These strategies will require the participation of stakeholders at the local, state, and national levels, including those in food production. Well-designed evaluation and research can guide future program improvements. The goal is a school meals environment in which students may choose from a variety of appealing and healthful options, leading to the consumption of foods that will promote their health and well-being.

1

Introduction and Background

This report provides recommendations targeted to improving two very large and important child nutrition programs overseen by the U.S. Department of Agriculture (USDA): namely, the National School Lunch Program (NSLP) and the School Breakfast Program (SBP). The school meal programs hold the potential to provide nearly all the nation's schoolchildren with access to nutritious, low-cost meals to support their growth, development, and health.

The purpose of the NSLP, as summarized in the 1946 enabling legislation, is "as a measure of national security, to safeguard the health and well-being of the Nation's children and to encourage the domestic consumption of nutritious agricultural commodities and other food" (*National School Lunch Act*, P.L. 79-396, Stat. 281 [June 4, 1946]: §2). Congress authorized the SBP as a pilot program in 1966 (*Child Nutrition Act*, P.L. 89-642 [October 11, 1966]). When Congress permanently authorized the SBP in 1975 under an amendment to the *Child Nutrition Act* (P.L. 94-105 [October 7, 1975]), it stated "it is the purpose and intent of the Congress that the school breakfast program be made available in all schools where it is needed to provide adequate nutrition for children in attendance" (Martin, 2008). Among the indications of need are large proportions of low-income children in the school and children who must travel long distances to school.

The potential reach of the school meal programs is very large: the NSLP is available in 99 percent of U.S. public schools and in 83 percent of private and public schools combined (USDA/ERS, 2004); the SBP is available in 85 percent of public schools (USDA/FNS, 2007a). If a school participates in one or both of the school meal programs, any child who attends the school may have access to the school meal. During the 2005–2006 school year, more than 49.1 million children were enrolled in U.S. public schools (U.S. Department of Education, 2007a).

In turn, about 60 percent of children in schools that offer school meals eat a lunch provided by the NSLP (USDA/FNS, 2007a). In fiscal year (FY) 2007, an average of 30.6 million schoolchildren participated in the NSLP on each school day. About 24 percent of children in schools that offered the SBP participated in the program, on average, equaling 10.1 million children each school day. In FY 2007, the participating schools served about 5.1 billion lunches at a federal cost of approximately $8.7 billion and 1.7 billion breakfasts at a federal cost of $2.2 billion (USDA/ERS, 2008a).

Both the NSLP and the SBP provide a safety net for children in need, given the provisions that make school meals available free or at a reduced cost to eligible participants. If the child lives in a household whose income is at or below 130 percent of the federal poverty level (or if the household receives food stamps,[1] Temporary Assistance for Needy Families, or assistance from the Food Distribution Program on Indian Reservations), the child is eligible for a free school lunch and a free school breakfast. The *McKinney-Vento Homeless Assistance Act* (P.L. 100-77 [1987]), as amended by the *No Child Left Behind Act* (P.L. 107-110 [2001]), states that students who are identified by a school district as homeless or highly mobile automatically qualify for free meals and do not need to complete the full application process (U.S. Department of Education, 2004).

A child is eligible for a reduced-price meal if the household income is between 130 and 185 percent of the poverty level (USDA/ERS, 2008b). Ordinarily, children from households with incomes over 185 percent of the poverty level pay full price. Even full-price meals, however, are subsidized by the government to a small extent through both cash reimbursements and the provision of USDA (commodity) foods (see Chapter 10).

Notably, in addition to providing food through the federal school meal programs, schools generally offer foods through à la carte service in the school cafeteria, school stores and snack bars, and vending machines. Food obtained from these sources and consumed at school is considered to be competitive food—food that competes with the school meal programs. Moreover, some schools have an open campus policy that gives students the opportunity to obtain food from commercial food establishments. The report *Nutrition Standards for Foods in Schools* (IOM, 2007a) recognizes that many of the competitive foods that are offered are not foods that are encouraged by the *Dietary Guidelines for Americans*. That report provides recommended standards for competitive foods to encourage students to

[1]As of October 1, 2008, the new name for the Food Stamp Program is the Supplemental Nutrition Assistance Program (commonly called SNAP).

consume foods that are healthful and to limit food components such as fats, added sugars, and sodium.

THE COMMITTEE'S TASK

USDA has sought the assistance of the Institute of Medicine (IOM) to provide recommendations to revise the nutrition- and food-related standards and requirements for the NSLP and the SBP. This request relates to the congressional requirement that USDA issue new guidance and regulations for the Nutrition Standards and Meal Requirements of the school meal programs (*Child Nutrition and WIC Reauthorization Act*, P.L. 108-265). The specific charge to the committee is shown in Box 1-1.

The committee's overall task was to review and assess the food and nutritional needs of schoolchildren in the United States on the basis of the 2005 *Dietary Guidelines for Americans* (HHS/USDA, 2005) and the Dietary Reference Intakes (DRIs) (IOM, 1997, 1998, 2000a, 2001, 2002/2005,

BOX 1-1
Charge to the Committee

- Specify a planning model for school meals (including targets for intake) as it may relate to nutrients and other dietary components for breakfast and lunch.

- Recommend revisions to the Nutrition Standards and, in consideration of the appropriate age-grade groups for schoolchildren, provide the calculations that quantify the amounts of nutrients and other dietary components specified in the Nutrition Standards.

- Recommend the Meal Requirements necessary to implement the Nutrition Standards on the basis of the two existing types of menu planning approaches (i.e., the food-based menu planning [FBMP] approach and the nutrient-based menu planning [NBMP] approach). The Meal Requirements are to include
  - standards for a food-based reimbursable meal by identifying
    – the food components for *as offered* and *as served* meals and
    – the amounts of food items per reimbursable meal by age-grade groups and
  - standards for a nutrient-based reimbursable meal by identifying
    – the menu items for *as offered* and *as served* and
    – the 5-day average amounts of nutrients and other dietary components per meal.

- Illustrate the practical application of the revised Nutrition Standards and Meal Requirements by developing 4 weeks of menus that will meet the recommended standards for the age-grade groups.

2005) and to use that review as a basis for recommending revisions to the Nutrition Standards and Meal Requirements for the NSLP and the SBP. As part of its task, the committee was asked to consider the critical issues identified by the Food and Nutrition Service (see Appendix C). The overall goal was the development of a set of well-conceived and practical recommendations for nutrients and Meal Requirements that reflect current nutrition science, increase the meals' contents of key food groups, improve the ability of the school meal programs to meet the nutritional needs of children, foster healthy eating habits, and safeguard children's health. The request to the committee specified that the recommendations be designed to be economical and to keep program costs as close as possible to current levels adjusted for inflation.

Current law requires the programs to provide meals containing one-third of the Recommended Dietary Allowance (RDA) for lunch and one-fourth of the RDA for breakfast. Congress adopted this language in 1994 before the development of the new conceptual approach and nutrient reference standards related to DRIs. Therefore, the committee's task included a request to compare differences (with examples and rationale) between basing standards on the RDA and basing the standards on values obtained using newer methods recommended by the IOM (2003).

The committee's work was divided into two phases. Phase I was completed with the release of the report *Nutrition Standards and Meal Requirements for the National School Lunch and Breakfast Programs: Phase I. Proposed Approach for Recommending Revisions* (IOM, 2008). That report covers the identification and review of the available data and information, the proposed criteria, an assessment of the food and nutrient intakes by schoolchildren, a description of the committee's planning model, and the analytic methods that it proposed to use to develop recommendations for revising the standards. Following the release of the Phase I report, the committee accepted comments from interested parties and held discussions of that report during a public workshop (see workshop agenda and a summary of public comments in Appendix D). This Phase II report builds on the Phase I effort and is the final report of the committee's work.

SCHOOL MEAL PROGRAMS OVERVIEW

Federal regulations have a major influence on the operation of the school meal programs and help to characterize them. To receive federal reimbursement, which accounts for a large share of the financial support for the programs, they are currently required to

- operate on a nonprofit basis,
- provide meals at no cost (free) or at a reduced price to children who qualify and are certified on the basis of household income,

- offer and serve meals that meet minimum nutrition standards and whose food components or menu items are consistent with program regulations, and
- meet *offer versus serve* (OVS) provisions of the *National School Lunch and Child Nutrition Act Amendment* (P.L. 94-105 [1975]) and subsequent amendments (P.L. 95-166, 97-35, 99-591). These provisions allow student choice as long as the number of items chosen meets the minimum specified by the *as served* standard. OVS is mandatory for senior high school meal programs and optional for the lower grades.

USDA establishes rates for reimbursement based on the number of qualifying meals served. In addition, using data on NSLP participation for the previous year, it sets a value for the commodity entitlement that the school districts may obtain.

The school meal programs are mistakenly believed by many to be mainly a USDA food distribution program. In reality, USDA foods account for only about 15 to 20 percent of the food served (USDA/FNS, 2008a). Concern has been expressed about the nutritional quality of USDA foods. However, great strides have been made: an increasing number of USDA foods can help the NSLP meet *Dietary Guidelines* and are highly acceptable to students (see Chapter 10).

Nutrition Standards and Meal Requirements

The program regulations that are the subject of this report are the Nutrition Standards and Meal Requirements. The elements of the current regulations pertaining to the Nutrition Standards and Meal Requirements are illustrated in Figure 1-1. The current planning model, which guided the development of the regulations, uses the 1995 *Dietary Guidelines for Americans* (HHS/USDA, 1995) and the 1989 RDAs (NRC, 1989).

The left-hand side of Figure 1-1 briefly describes each of the elements of the school meal process, and the right-hand side shows how the elements are connected to provide a pathway to a nutritious school breakfast or lunch. Under the OVS provision, the child's selections are out of the direct control of the provider. Consumption of the food is a key part of ensuring the health of children, but it is out of the direct control of the meal's providers as well. Although it is desirable that Nutrition Standards and Meal Requirements take into account the acceptability of meals to students to the extent possible, key factors that affect students' selection and consumption of the food, such as the environment in which the meals are served and the quality of the food served, are beyond the scope of this report.

The Nutrition Standards provide the health foundation for the NSLP and the SBP. The related Meal Requirements facilitate the actions needed to implement the Nutrition Standards and develop menus and meals. At

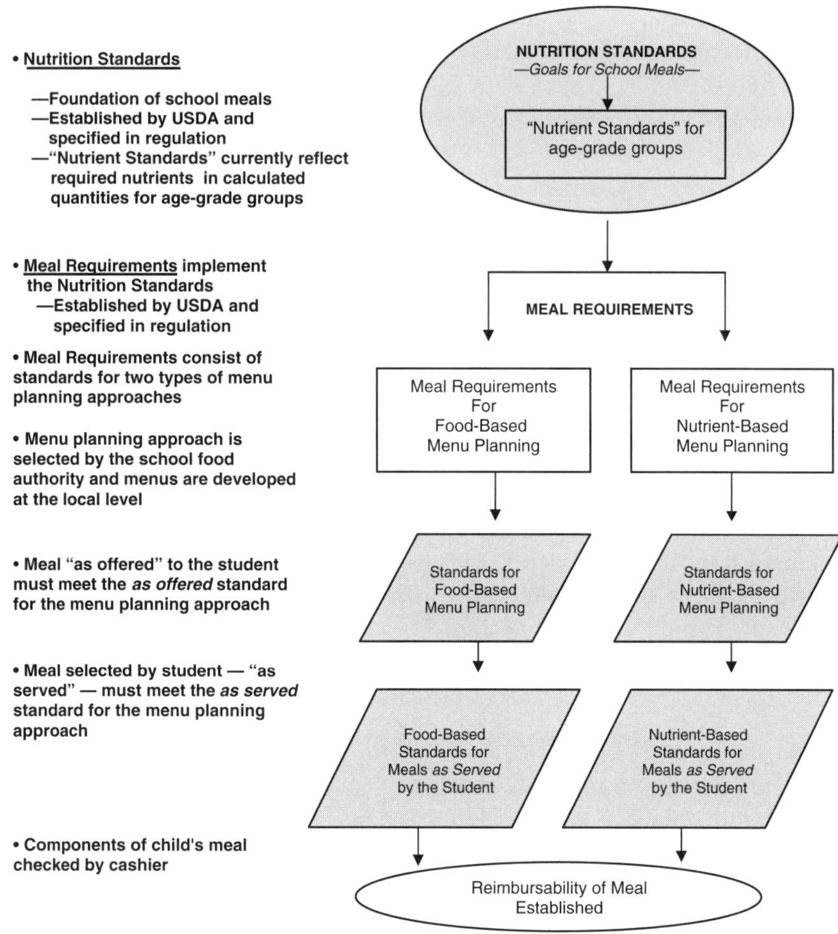

FIGURE 1-1 Relationships among *current* Nutrition Standards, Meal Requirements, and eligibility for federal reimbursement.

present, Meal Requirements include meal standards for two general types of menu planning approaches:[2]

[2]There actually are two categories of the food-based approach (traditional and enhanced), two categories of the nutrient-based approach (nutrient standard menu planning and assisted nutrient standard menu planning), and a fifth option (any reasonable approach) (see USDA/FNS [2007b] for details).

1. the food-based menu planning (FBMP) approach, which focuses on the types and the amounts of foods to be offered to meet the Nutrition Standards; and
2. the nutrient-based menu planning (NBMP) approach, which makes use of computer software to plan menus that meet the Nutrition Standards.

Local school food authorities[3] (SFAs) decide which menu planning approach to use and, hence, which set of meal standards is to be followed. Currently, approximately 70 percent of schools use the FBMP approach (USDA/FNS, 2007a). Existing meal standards for the two most common types of menu planning (the traditional approach and the nutrient standard menu planning approach) appear in Appendix E.

Figure 1-2 identifies the standards that are the main focus of the committee's task and illustrates their interrelationships. The committee's task requires that its recommendations for new Nutrition Standards be consistent with the current (2005) *Dietary Guidelines for Americans* and with current nutrient reference values and methods of applying them. As noted earlier and shown in Figure 1-2, the Nutrition Standards apply equally regardless of the meal planning approach used.

Description of the Current Nutrition Standards

The *Healthy Meals for Healthy Americans Act of 1994* (P.L. 103-448, Sec. 106(b)) requires that the Nutrition Standards of the NSLP and the SBP meals remain consistent with the most recent the *Dietary Guidelines for Americans*. Current regulations used the 1995 *Dietary Guidelines for Americans* to specify a minimum and maximum for the amount of total fat and a maximum for the amount of saturated fat. Legislation passed in 1996 (*Personal Responsibility and Work Opportunity Reconciliation Act of 1996*, P.L. 104-193 [August 22, 1996]) mandated that school meals provide on average, over a 5-day week, at least

- (school lunch) one-third of the RDA of the Food and Nutrition Board, and
- (school breakfast) one-fourth of the RDA.

The law does not specify the nutrients to be included.

[3]Local school food authorities encompass school districts or small groups of districts that are approved by the USDA Food and Nutrition Service to operate the school meal programs (USDA/FNS, 2007b).

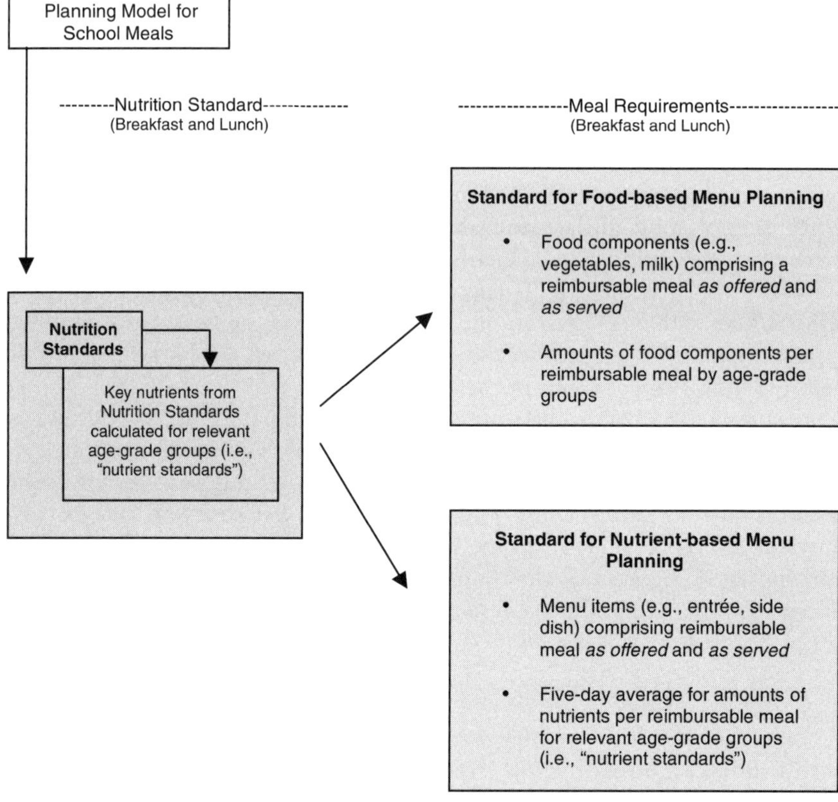

FIGURE 1-2 Current standards for school breakfast and lunch under review by the committee.

The existing USDA regulations cover calories[4] and five nutrients that are to be provided by school meals. The five nutrients were chosen because of the roles they play in promoting growth and development (USDA/FNS, 1995), and they were intended to serve as a practical proxy for other nutrients. The Nutrition Standards specify the minimum amounts of calories and the five nutrients and the maximum amount of saturated fat for selected age-grade groups (e.g., grades 7–12). The Nutrition Standards also list the recommended (but not required) levels of cholesterol, sodium, and dietary fiber in the school meals. These nutrients and the other dietary components

[4]The term *calories* is used to refer to kilocalories throughout this report.

are identified on the nutrition labels of food products, providing an important source of information for school menu planners.

Description of Meal Requirements

Existing Meal Requirements differ depending on which menu planning approach is chosen by the SFA. The Meal Requirements lay out standards for reimbursable meals as they are *offered* to students and, under the OVS provision of the law, as they are *served* to students.[5] Tables 1-1 and 1-2 summarize the standards for reimbursable meals *as offered* and *as served* for the two general types of meal planning approach. Details on the amounts of foods may be found in *The Road to SMI Success: A Guide for Food Service Directors* (USDA/FNS, 2007b).

Under the OVS provision (USDA/FNS, 1976), which is mandatory at the high school level, a student may select (be served) fewer menu items than must be offered. For the selected meal to be reimbursable, however, the number of selections must match the number specified in the *as served* standard. For example, as indicated in Table 1-1 for food-based menu planning, a lunch selected by a high school student that consisted of one serving of fluid milk, one serving of meat or meat alternate, one serving of grain/bread, and no servings of fruits and vegetables would be reimbursable. In nutrient-based menu planning, a lunch that included only the entrée and one side dish (for example) would be reimbursable.

REASONS FOR THE UPDATING OF NUTRITION STANDARDS AND MEAL REQUIREMENTS

Congressional Mandate

In recognition of the need to update and revise the Nutrition Standards and Meal Requirements for the school meal programs, Congress incorporated requirements in the 2004 *Child Nutrition and WIC*[6] *Reauthorization Act* (P.L. 108-265). In particular, the act requires USDA to issue guidance and regulations to promote the consistency of the standards for school meal programs with the standards provided in the most recent *Dietary Guidelines for Americans* and DRIs. A new edition of the *Dietary Guidelines* and the complete set of DRIs, both of which encourage intakes of foods and

[5]In schools in which the OVS provision is not in effect (some elementary and middle schools), the standard is that the student must make a selection of each type of food components or menu item.

[6]WIC is the Special Supplemental Nutrition Program for Women, Infants, and Children.

TABLE 1-1 Reimbursable School Meals Planned Using a Food-Based Approach: Standards for Food Components *as Offered* and *as Served*, by Type of Meal

Meal	*As Offered*	*As Served*
Breakfast[a]	• One fluid milk • One vegetable/fruit • Two meat/meat alternates; two grain/bread; or one meat/meat alternate and one grain/bread (Total of four items)	Students must select three of the four items[b]
Lunch[c]	• One fluid milk • One meat/meat alternate • Two vegetables/fruit • One grain/bread (Total of five items)	Senior high school level: students must select three of the five items Grades below senior high school level: students must select either three or four of the five items

[a]The minimum amount of food that must be offered is the same from kindergarten through grade 12, except that an additional serving of any of the grains or breads is optional for students in grades 7 through 12 under the enhanced food-based approach; the range is shown in Appendix Table E-1.

[b]*Offer versus serve* for breakfast is optional at all grade levels.

[c]The minimum amounts of food that must be offered depend on the age-grade group and the approach (traditional or enhanced).

SOURCE: Derived from USDA/FNS, 2007b.

TABLE 1-2 Reimbursable Breakfast and Lunch Planned Using a Nutrient-Based Approach: Standards for Menu Items *as Offered* and *as Served*, by Type of Meal

Meal	*As Offered*	*As Served*
Breakfast[a]	Schools must offer at least three menu items: • Fluid milk (served as a beverage) • Two additional menu items	• Student may decline only one item, regardless of the number of items offered
Lunch[b]	Schools must offer at least three menu items: • Fluid milk • Entrée • Side dish	• If three items are offered, students may decline one • If four or more items are offered, students may decline two • Students must select an entrée

[a]*Offer versus serve* (OVS) for breakfast is optional at all grade levels.

[b]OVS is optional in grades below senior high level.

SOURCE: Derived from USDA/FNS, 2007b.

nutrients that have been associated with good health and chronic disease prevention, were released after the latest set of Nutrition Standards and Meal Requirements regulations had become effective.

In response to the congressional mandate, USDA has updated some of its materials for food service professionals to include information on the 2005 *Dietary Guidelines for Americans*. For example, the *Menu Planner for Healthy School Meals* (USDA/FNS, 2008b) includes a description of the 2005 *Dietary Guidelines for Americans* and guidance on how to implement them in school programs. *Fact Sheets for Healthier School Meals* includes guidance on preparing and serving meals consistent with the *Dietary Guidelines* (USDA/FNS, 2009a).

Consistency with Dietary Guidelines for Americans

Among the changes needed to improve consistency with the 2005 edition of *Dietary Guidelines for Americans* are the following:

- Increasing the emphasis on food groups to encourage a healthier food consumption pattern, especially by offering variety and a larger amount of fruits and vegetables, and by offering whole grains as a substitute for some refined grains, and
- Limiting the intake of saturated fat, *trans* fat, cholesterol, added sugars, and salt by offering foods such as fat-free (skim) milk or low-fat milk, fewer sweetened foods, and foods with little added salt.

Consistency with Dietary Reference Intakes

The DRI values and the recommended approaches for applying them produce a markedly different basis for the Nutrition Standards than do the 1989 RDAs (the reference values on which the existing Nutrition Standards are based). The DRIs cover many more nutrients and include four types of reference values (see Chapter 3 for details). The DRIs are "intended to help individuals optimize their health, prevent disease, and avoid consuming too much of a nutrient" (IOM, 2006, p. 1). For groups of people, such as school-aged children, the aim of the DRI values is to achieve usual intake *distributions* for nutrients such that (1) the prevalence of intakes that are inadequate is low and (2) the prevalence of intakes at risk of being excessive also is low. Chapter 7 provides comparative information related to possible Nutrition Standards based on the RDAs and those set using methods recommended by the IOM (2003).

Other Considerations

Ease of Implementation of Regulations

The implementation of the current Nutrition Standards and Meal Requirements poses challenges for many school food operators and their schools (IOM, 2008). The Food and Nutrition Service and other stakeholders have called for a simplification of the meal planning regulations for reimbursable meals. The committee addresses ease of implementation in its methods of developing the Meal Requirements (Chapters 5 and 6) and in its discussion of implementing the recommendations in Chapter 10.

Children's Health and Well-Being

Currently, overweight and obesity are major health concerns for the nation's children (CDC, 2008; Ogden et al., 2008). The development of recommendations for Nutrition Standards and Meal Requirements for school meals must consider evidence related to the promotion of growth and development and a healthy weight. At the same time, the school meal programs play a key role in helping to alleviate food insecurity and inadequate intakes. The recommended standards will need to achieve an appropriate balance—that is, avoiding excessive calories while allowing for enough appropriate calories and nutrients to support the needs of those children with inadequate intakes.

REVISED TERMINOLOGY

In the course of its work, the committee determined that a new term was needed to accurately represent its recommendations. In particular, the committee developed recommendations for *Nutrient Targets* rather than Nutrition Standards. The rationale for the change in terminology appears in Chapter 4. This new term appears below where applicable in the description of the organization of the report.

SUMMARY AND ORGANIZATION OF THE REPORT

The school meal programs help guard the health and well-being of the nation's children, in large part through the implementation of a complex set of Nutrition Standards and Meal Requirements. Congress mandated an update of the Nutrition Standards and Meal Requirements following the release of new scientific evidence in *Dietary Guidelines for Americans* (HHS/USDA, 2005) and in a series of reports on DRIs (IOM, 1997, 1998, 2000a, 2000b, 2001, 2002/2005, 2003, 2005).

The overall goal of the committee was the development of a set of well-conceived, practical, and economical recommendations for updating the current Nutrition Standards and Meal Requirements—recommendations that reflect current nutrition and health science, increase the meals' contents of specified food groups, and improve the ability of the school meal programs to meet the nutritional needs of children, foster healthy eating habits, and safeguard children's health.

The following chapters describe the processes used by the committee to meet that goal and present its findings, conclusions, and recommendations. Chapter 2 lays the foundation for revising the Nutrition Standards and Meal Requirements. Chapter 3 describes children's food and nutrient intakes and identifies possible areas of concern. Chapters 4 and 5 describe the processes used to develop the Nutrient Targets and Meal Requirements, respectively. Chapter 6 provides perspective on the iterative nature of the processes and on challenges that confronted the committee. Chapter 7 presents the recommendations for Nutrient Targets and Meal Requirements. Subsequent chapters cover food cost and market effects; the projected impact of the recommended Nutrient Targets and Meal Requirements; and recommendations for implementation (including monitoring), evaluation, and research.

2

Foundation for Revising Nutrition Standards and Meal Requirements

To provide a firm foundation for revising the Nutrition Standards and Meal Requirements, the committee carefully considered its overall approach and major challenges, which are summarized here. In addition, this chapter presents the rationale for (1) establishing three age-grade groups representing elementary school, middle school, and high school and (2) setting mean values for the total daily calorie requirements for those age-grade groups, which have been rounded to 1,800, 2,000, and 2,400 calories, respectively.

THE APPROACH

The committee's approach to developing recommendations for revisions to the Nutrition Standards and Meal Requirements for the School Breakfast Program and the National School Lunch Program included numerous steps. The committee

1. Developed and applied a set of working principles to guide the selection of evidence and the types of analyses and reviews to be conducted and to focus committee deliberations. The working principles, shown in Box 2-1, were developed during Phase I and applied throughout the study.
2. Developed a set of criteria to assist in deriving and evaluating the recommendations. These criteria, shown in Box 2-2, were developed during Phase I and slightly revised during Phase II in response to feedback on the Phase I report (IOM, 2008).

BOX 2-1
Working Principles for Determining Recommendations for Revisions to the Nutrition Standards and Meal Requirements for School Meals

1. The present and future health and well-being of schoolchildren are profoundly affected by their food and nutrient intakes and the maintenance of healthy body weight.

a. School meals, when they are consumed, should improve food and nutrient intakes, and those intakes that are inadequate or excessive in school-aged children should specifically be targeted.

b. School meals are targeted to children ages 4 through 18 years, but younger children and children of all ages with special needs may be affected by the standards set for the general population.

c. Recognition will be given to health effects of foods (including beverages) that go beyond those related to their nutrient content.

2. School breakfast and lunch programs, which may contribute to more than 50 percent of the caloric intake by children on school days, offer opportunities to promote the health and well-being of children.

a. School meals can contribute to beneficial health and dietary patterns and are uniquely positioned to provide a model for healthy meals and to provide opportunities to model and reinforce healthy eating behaviors.

b. School meals can provide a platform for education in nutrition, environmental responsibility, and food safety.

c. School meals can be a positive environment for pleasant social interactions.

d. For children in families characterized by limited resources and food insecurity, school meals provide a critical safety net in meeting their nutritional needs and reducing the adverse effects of food insecurity.

3. School breakfast and lunch programs operate in a challenging and changing environment.

a. School food service environments (such as facilities, equipment, labor, and skills) are complex and highly varied across the nation as well as from school to school within school districts.

b. Challenges include the need to meet food safety standards, offer appetizing foods to an increasingly diverse population, adjust to the changes in the available food supply, improve the image and appeal of the program, and achieve a sound financial operation.

c. Food costs, other direct costs, and indirect costs related to program operation are outpacing the available resources.

d. In addition to promoting the health and well-being of children, high rates of participation may support the financial stability of school meal programs.

e. Efforts to change the current school nutrition environments vary, with some districts already making significant strides and others just starting the process of change.

4. Because scientific findings and authoritative recommendations related to the nutrition of children evolve over time, the process of developing recommendations for revisions should be transparent and designed to take into account new evidence-based findings and recommendations.

BOX 2-2
Criteria for the Nutrient Targets and Meal Requirements for the School Breakfast Program and the National School Lunch Program

Criterion 1. The Nutrient Targets and Meal Requirements are consistent with current dietary guidance and nutrition recommendations to promote health—as exemplified by the *Dietary Guidelines for Americans* and the Dietary Reference Intakes—with the ultimate goal of improving children's diets by reducing the prevalence of inadequate and excessive intakes of food, nutrients, and calories.

Criterion 2. The Nutrient Targets and Meal Requirements will be considered on the basis of age-grade groups that are consistent with the current age-gender categories used for specifying reference values and with widely used school grade configurations.

Criterion 3. The Nutrient Targets and Meal Requirements will result in the simplification of the menu planning and monitoring processes, and they will be compatible with the development of menus that are practical to prepare and serve and that offer nutritious foods and beverages that appeal to students of diverse cultural backgrounds.

Criterion 4. The Nutrient Targets and Meal Requirements will be sensitive to program costs and school administrative concerns.

3. Set key parameters including age-grade groups and total daily mean calorie requirements for each group. The methods used to set these parameters are described later in this chapter.

4. Assessed schoolchildren's dietary intakes and considered relevant laboratory data and health effects of inadequate or excessive intakes. Dietary intakes included food groups, food subgroups, energy, and nutrients. The purpose was to identify the food and nutrient intakes of concern for specified age-grade groups. Chapter 3 covers this topic.

5. Examined and tested various approaches for developing the Nutrient Targets, including energy targets. The committee used methods recommended by the Institute of Medicine (IOM, 2003) when applicable. Chapter 4 covers this topic.

6. Determined that only one approach to meal planning would be recommended and that the Nutrient Targets would be the scientific basis of the standards for menu planning, but they would be only one of the elements considered when developing these standards. Chapter 5 covers the development of the Meal Requirements.

7. Using an iterative approach (described in Chapter 6), applied the criteria listed in Box 2-2 to finalize the committee's recommendations for the Nutrient Targets and Meal Requirements, giving special emphasis to

the practicality of the Meal Requirements. Chapter 7 presents the recommendations. In applying the criteria, the committee considered

- the food cost implications of the recommended revisions (see Chapter 8) and
- the effects of various assumptions on potential nutrition-related outcomes (see Chapter 9).

In addition, the committee addressed potential market effects of the recommended revisions. This content is covered in Chapter 8.

As a result of the committee's process and decisions, a new figure was needed to illustrate the recommended elements in the pathway to a nutritious school meal (see Figure 2-1).

Figure 2-2 illustrates the complex nature of the process used by the committee to revise the Nutrition Standards and Meal Requirements for the school meal programs. The first box that addresses Nutrient Targets, for example, indicates that methods need to be developed for setting those targets. The boxes on either side that specify considering or evaluating specific elements relate to the application of the committee's criteria. The double arrows and dashed lines indicate the iterative steps in the process. For example, initial proposals for the Meal Requirements were tested to determine how well they aligned with the committee's criteria, and the results were used to modify the proposals to achieve a better fit. Extensive analyses provided the foundation for the recommendations. The major product of the process was a set of recommendations for Nutrient Targets and Meal Requirements.

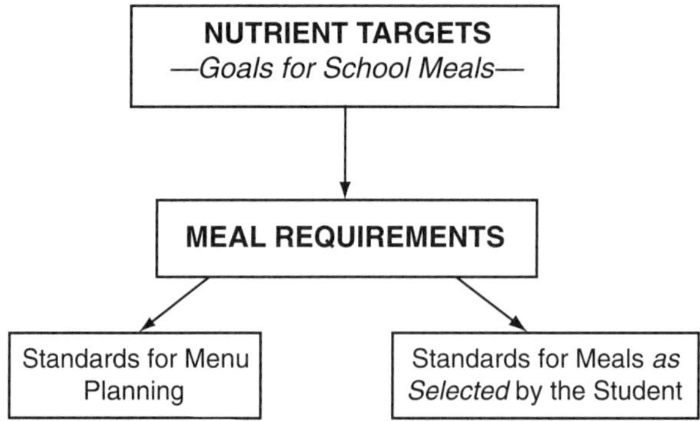

FIGURE 2-1 Depiction of the *recommended* elements in the path to nutritious school meals. In this figure and throughout the remainder of the report, the committee uses the term *as selected by the student* (or simply *as selected*) rather than *as served* to apply to standards for reimbursable meals.

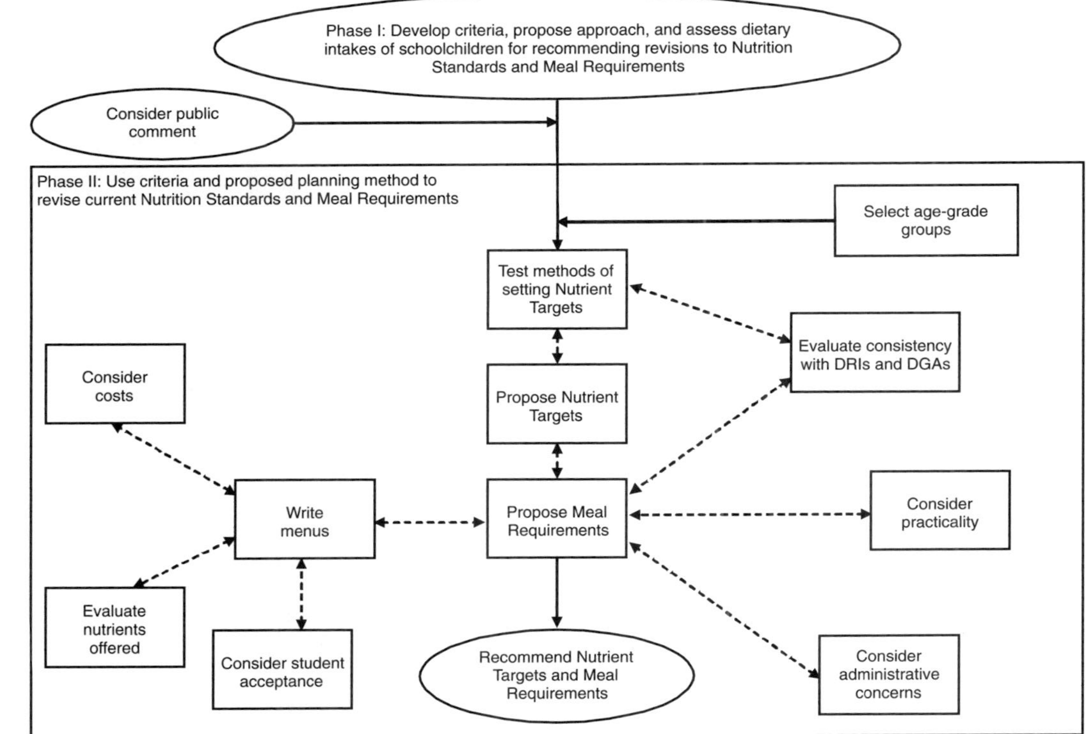

FIGURE 2-2 Process for revising current Nutrition Standards and Meal Requirements for the National School Lunch and the School Breakfast Programs. Dashed lines indicate the iterative nature of the process.
NOTES: DGA = *Dietary Guidelines for Americans*; DRI = Dietary Reference Intakes.

MAJOR CHALLENGES IN APPLYING GROUP PLANNING APPROACHES FOR SCHOOL MEALS

For some decisions, especially those focused on applying recommendations given in *Dietary Guidelines for Americans* (HHS/USDA, 2005), the process for setting Nutrient Targets was straightforward. The application of Dietary Reference Intakes (DRIs) to inform the decision-making process, however, was quite complex.

A report by the IOM (2003) lays out a framework for using DRIs to plan nutrient intakes for groups. The DRI process involves "identifying the specific nutritional goals, determining how best to achieve these goals, and, ultimately, assessing if these goals are achieved" (IOM, 2003, p. 7). According to the framework, the overall goal is "to determine a distribution of usual nutrient intakes that provides for a low prevalence of inadequate intakes and a low prevalence of intakes that may be at potential risk of adverse effects due to excessive intake" (IOM, 2003, p. 8). The IOM report provides scientifically based guidance for selecting the specific goals for different kinds of groups but acknowledges that research is needed on techniques and other aspects of group planning.

Using the DRI framework to develop Nutrient Targets and Meal Requirements for school meals poses a number of challenges. The major challenges include the following:

- Any age-grade grouping of schoolchildren is very heterogeneous in terms of the calorie and nutrient needs of the members of the group (consider, for example, small sedentary adolescent females and large adolescent male athletes). The methods for planning for heterogeneous groups covered in *Dietary Reference Intakes: Applications in Dietary Planning* (IOM, 2003) are described as based on theory rather than on evidence and are in need of further research. This school meals report presents one of the first applications of methods recommended by the IOM for developing targets for planning meals. The applications differ somewhat from those used by an earlier committee to develop recommendations for revision of the food packages for the Supplemental Nutrition Program for Women, Infants, and Children (WIC) (IOM, 2005).
- The children who participate in one or more school meal programs obtain only a part of their daily intake from the school meal(s). To estimate changes in total daily intake and the resulting changes in the prevalence of inadequate and excessive intakes, an assumption must be made about how changes in the school meals will affect intake at other eating occasions.
- The relationship of Nutrient Targets to children's food and nutrient consumption is complex. Schoolchildren's food selections affect their actual intake. School meal programs typically offer children a range of choices

within menu item categories (e.g., a choice of milks, a choice of entrées), and the *offer versus serve* provision of the law allows children to refuse some of the foods that must be offered (e.g., they may decline to take a milk or a grain). In addition, children may not eat all the food they select. Chapters 6 and 7 address this topic in detail.

The nature of these challenges highlights the importance of the third step in the DRI process: "assessing if these goals are achieved." Such assessment can occur only after implementation of the Nutrient Targets and Meal Requirements and thus is beyond the scope of this committee's work. Nonetheless, such assessments must occur and their outcomes serve as the basis for future enhancements of the school meal programs. The focus of related research is outlined in Chapter 10 of this report.

DEFINING KEY PARAMETERS: AGE-GRADE GROUPS AND ENERGY REQUIREMENTS

Establishing Age-Grade Groups

Establishing age-grade groups of schoolchildren was the first step in the formulation of the Nutrition Standards and Meal Requirements. The U.S. Department of Agriculture (USDA) asked the committee to recommend age-grade groups that reflect the stages of growth and development in children and adolescents.

Currently, the age groupings for the Nutrient Targets are based in part on age groupings in the 1989 Recommended Dietary Allowances (NRC, 1989). Current Meal Requirements for the School Breakfast Program specify one grade range—kindergarten through grade 12—regardless of the menu planning approach being used. However, some menu planning approaches include a breakfast option for grades 7 through 12 that allows somewhat more food for these older children. Current Meal Requirements for the National School Lunch Program are set for an array of grade groupings,[1] which differ by the type of menu planning approach used (USDA/FNS, 2007b).

To determine the most appropriate age-grade groups, the committee considered two major elements:

1. evidence on current school grade spans and grade organization trends and

---

[1]Excluding preschool, the current groupings for lunch are kindergarten through grade 3, kindergarten through grade 6, grades 4 through 12, and grades 7 through 12.

2. the DRI age categories for school-aged children (4–8 years, 9–13 years, and 14–18 years).

Grade Organizations

Data from the National Center for Education Statistics (U.S. Department of Education, 2007b) indicate that the most common grade organizational plan in school districts throughout the nation has three tiers. The plans vary somewhat but typically encompass elementary school (kindergarten or grade 1 through grades 5 or 6), middle school (grades 5 or 6 through grade 8) (U.S. Department of Education, 2000), and high school (grades 9 through 12). McEwin et al. (2003) report that since the 1970s there has been a steady movement from a two-tier plan (e.g., grades kindergarten through 8 and grades 9 through 12) to a three-tier plan, most commonly grades kindergarten through 5, 6 through 8, and 9 through 12. The U.S. Department of Education (2000) reports that nearly all the new middle schools served children in grades 6 through 8.

Comparison of Dietary Reference Intake Age Groups with Grade Organizations

The DRI age groups are based on biological evidence about children's development (IOM, 1997). The committee considered how the ages of children included in the three most common grade spans (grades kindergarten through 5, 6 through 8, and 9 through 12) compare with DRI age groupings (Table 2-1). It concluded that the three grade spans in Table 2-1 would provide the basis for practical yet developmentally appropriate age-grade groupings for use in developing the Nutrient Targets and Meal Requirements. The kindergarten through grade 5 group received special attention because it includes children from two DRI age groups.

In conclusion, the most practical and developmentally appropriate age-grade groups for use in developing the Nutrient Targets and Meal Requirements are as follows:

Type of School	Age Range (years)	Grade Range
Elementary school	5–10	Kindergarten through 5
Middle school	11–13	6 through 8
High school	14–18	9 through 12

These age-grade groupings were used in setting the Nutrient Targets and the standards for menu planning.

TABLE 2-1 Age Spans for Typical Grade Organizations Compared with Age Ranges for Dietary Reference Intakes

Grade Span	Typical Age Span for the Grade Span[a] (years)	Corresponding DRI Age Ranges[b] (years)
K–5	5–10 or 11	4–8 and 9–13
6–8	11–13 or 14	9–13
9–12	14–18	14–18

NOTES: DRI = Dietary Reference Intakes; K = kindergarten; y = years.
SOURCES: [a]U.S. Department of Education, 2001; [b]IOM, 1997.

Estimated Energy Requirements

To set Nutrient Targets for school meals it is essential to determine appropriate estimates of average daily energy requirements by age-grade group—values that are applied to both the males and females in the group. Of necessity, these values will be too high for some children (mainly the youngest elementary schoolchildren and the adolescent females) and too low for others. Using the methods described below, the committee sought to achieve a satisfactory balance.

Energy requirements for males and females ages 5 through 18 years were estimated using the age- and gender-specific Estimated Energy Requirement equations in *Dietary Reference Intakes: Energy, Carbohydrate, Fiber, Fat, Fatty Acids, Cholesterol, Protein, and Amino Acids* (IOM, 2002/2005). To apply these equations, the committee needed to specify the height and weight of males and females ages 5 through 18 years and to make assumptions regarding their physical activity level. The values selected and the rationale for their selection are provided below.

Height and Weight Adjustments

Three sources of data on the height and weight of school-aged children were considered: (1) the 2000 Centers for Disease Control and Prevention (CDC) growth charts (Kuczmarski et al., 2000), (2) the National Health and Nutrition Examination Survey (NHANES) covering 1999–2004 (Personal communication, Dr. Nancy Cole and Mary Kay Fox, Mathematica Policy Research, Inc., March 2009), and (3) the third School Nutrition Dietary Assessment study (SNDA-III) that collected data during the 2004–2005 school year (USDA/FNS, 2007a). Ultimately, the committee decided to use median heights and weights from the 2000 CDC growth charts because they are the reference standards for healthy U.S. children. Both the NHANES 1999–2004 data and the SNDA-III data were ruled out because of higher median weights and higher prevalence of obesity, relative to the

CDC reference standards, reflecting recent increases in obesity among U.S. youth. For a similar reason, the CDC did not use data from NHANES-III (1988–1994) when updating the growth charts in the late 1990s (IOM, 2002/2005).

Physical Activity Level Assumptions

To calculate the Estimated Energy Requirement, one needs an estimate of an individual's usual physical activity level (PAL). Self-report methods of estimating a child's physical activity, such as physical activity questionnaires or diaries, have low validity (Adamo et al., 2009; Corder et al., 2008; Janz et al., 1995; Sallis and Saelens, 2000). Therefore, to assign a PAL to school-aged children, the committee relied mainly on available accelerometry data.

Physical Activity Level of U.S. Children Accelerometers (physical activity monitors) are small electronic devices programmed to detect and record the magnitude of accelerations of the body. The chief advantage of accelerometers over self-report methods is that they provide an objective measure of engagement in physical activity. Also, the magnitude (intensity) of an activity may be captured on a minute-by-minute basis, thereby providing a better measure of engagement in moderate and vigorous physical activities than is possible with a self-report questionnaire.

The committee reviewed accelerometer data from a number of studies (Janz et al., 2005; McMurray et al., 2008; Nader et al., 2008; Troiano et al., 2008; Troped et al., 2007; Whitt-Glover et al., 2009). However, the only accelerometer data that were used by the committee were collected as part of the 2003–2004 NHANES[2] and analyzed by Troiano et al. (2008). None of the other studies collected data on a nationally representative sample of children. Rather, most involved cohort or convenience samples of children in one geographic area or several regions, males or females only, or children within a narrow age range (e.g., middle school children). Nonetheless, with only one exception (Nader et al., 2008), the results of the less representative studies were fairly consistent with the NHANES results. Using the same NHANES data set used by Troiano and colleagues (2008), Whitt-Glover and coworkers (2009) found no significant differences in physical activity by socioeconomic status.

The analysis of the NHANES accelerometer data provided estimates of the average number of minutes per day that Americans spend engaged in moderate and vigorous intensity physical activities. Table 2-2 presents the

[2]A detailed description of the NHANES physical activity monitor procedures may be found at http://www.cdc.gov/nchs/nhanes/nhanes2003-2004/exam03_04.htm.

TABLE 2-2 Mean Minutes per Day of Engagement in Moderate or Vigorous Physical Activity,* NHANES 2003–2004

Age (years)	Males (min/d)[a]	PAL Classification[b]	Females (min/d)[a]	PAL Classification[b]
6–11	95.4	Active	75.2	Active
12–15	45.3	Low active	24.6	Sedentary
16–19	32.7	Low active	19.6	Sedentary

NOTES: min/d = minutes per day; NHANES = National Health and Nutrition Examination Survey; PAL = physical activity level.

*Minutes of vector magnitude readings indicative of engagement in moderate or vigorous physical activity based on age-specific criteria.

SOURCES: [a]Troiano et al., 2008; [b]IOM, 2002/2005.

TABLE 2-3 Physical Activity Level Category Classifications Used to Calculate Estimated Energy Requirements of School-Aged Children, by Age and Gender

Ages (years)	Males	Females
6–10	Active	Active
11–13	Low active	Low active
14–18	Low active	Low active

mean minutes per day that U.S. children were found to be engaged in moderate or vigorous physical activities and the PAL categories that correspond with each. To summarize the results, for most age and gender groups, the average total daily minutes of engagement in moderate or vigorous activities fit within the *active* or *low active* categories. However, the average total daily minutes of engagement in moderate or vigorous activity for females ages 12–15 and 16–19 years fit within the *sedentary* activity category.

Physical Activity Level Categories The PAL categories the committee selected for use in estimating the energy requirements of males and females of various ages are presented in Table 2-3.[3] For young males of all ages and females ages 5–10 years, the categories selected match those indicated by the NHANES 2003–2004 accelerometer data (Table 2-2). However, for females ages 11–13 and 14–18 years, the committee determined that a low active rather than a sedentary category of classification was warranted for use in the calculation of the Estimated Energy Requirements for two reasons:

[3]The committee recognizes that the data summarized in Table 2-2 are for somewhat different age groups but considers them close enough to use as a basis for PALs.

1. Public health measures call for at least a low-active level of physical activity for children of school age.

2. Calorie levels need to be high enough to allow for planning school meals that meet an appropriate portion of schoolchildrens' food and nutrient needs.

The assumption of the low-active PAL resulted in Estimated Energy Requirements for the females in the two older age-grade groups that are about 20 percent higher than would be calculated using a sedentary physical activity level. When the Estimated Energy Requirements for the males and females are averaged, however, the result is only about 8 percent higher. Furthermore, offering a small amount of extra calories may be justified for the adolescents because the range between the male and female calorie requirements is large (especially for the high school ages). Thus, the active boys may need the additional calories, while the inactive girls would have the option to choose or to consume less.

Information about how these classifications were used in the calculation of the Estimated Energy Requirements for males and females of school age appears in Appendix F.

Mean Estimated Energy Requirements

The Estimated Energy Requirements determined by the process described above appear in Appendix F. The *mean* Estimated Energy Requirement was then calculated by gender and by age-grade group (5–10 years for kindergarten through grade 5, 11–13 years for grades 6 through 8, and 14–18 years for grades 9 through 12). The calculated mean daily calorie requirements for males and females by age-grade group appear in Table 2-4.

TABLE 2-4 Calculated Mean Daily Calorie Requirements[a] by Age-Grade Group for Males and Females Separately and for Both Genders Combined

	Calories (kcal)		
Age-Grade Group	Males	Females	Males and Females Combined
Ages 5–10 years, Kindergarten–Grade 5	1,894	1,765	1,829
Ages 11–13 years, Grade 6–8	2,125	1,905	2,015
Ages 14–18 years, Grade 9–12	2,686	2,044	2,365

NOTE: y = years.

[a]These requirements were obtained from the mean Estimated Energy Requirement calculations for the age-grade-gender group.

The committee used these mean daily calorie levels by gender and age-grade group when setting the preliminary nutrient targets for vitamins, minerals, and protein (see Chapter 4). Rounded mean daily calorie levels for both genders combined (1,800, 2,000, and 2,400 calories) were used in calculations to set minimum and maximum calorie targets for school meals (see Chapter 4) and in calculations related to the Meal Requirements.

SUMMARY

The committee used a seven-step approach to the design of Nutrient Targets and Meal Requirements. The major challenges identified are the need to work with complex interrelationships among heterogeneous groupings of children for whom school meals provide only part of their nutritional intake and for whom food preferences differ. Data-based methods were used to provide a basis for two key decisions that were critical to the development of recommended Nutrient Targets and Meal Requirements: the setting of age-grade groups for school meals and the calculation of appropriate values for mean total daily calorie requirements for males and females in those age groups. The age-grade groups chosen were 5–10 years (kindergarten through grade 5), 11–13 years (grades 6 through 8), and 14–18 years (grades 9 through 12). Subsequent chapters address the assessment of schoolchildren's dietary intakes, other data related to the children's nutritional health, the development of the Nutrient Targets and Meal Requirements, various analyses, and recommendations and guidance for implementation.

3

Schoolchildren's Food and Nutrient Intakes and Related Health Concerns

PRÉCIS

This chapter summarizes key information about schoolchildren's reported food and nutrient intakes, and it also covers supportive findings that influenced the committee's decision-making process for developing recommended Nutrient Targets and Meal Requirements for the school meal programs. Several undesirable aspects of children's intakes were identified. Of special note are low mean daily intakes of fruits, vegetables (especially dark green and orange vegetables and legumes), and whole grains as well as high intakes of discretionary calories (calories mainly from solid fat and added sugars) and sodium. Adolescent females tended to have low reported intakes of nearly all the nutrients investigated by the committee.

BACKGROUND

The committee assessed the dietary intakes of food groups, food subgroups, and nutrients by schoolchildren to identify food and nutrient intakes of concern by age-grade group and provide key information needed to develop recommendations for Nutrient Targets and Meal Requirements. The data sources and methods used by the committee are outlined below. The Phase I report (IOM, 2008) provides a detailed description of the data sources and methods, and Appendix G of this final report includes tables covering new analyses for schoolchildren's intakes of energy and of magnesium to illustrate the type of data generated for the committee. The two major sources of food and nutrient data used were (1) *Diet*

Quality of American School-Age Children by School Lunch Participation Status (USDA/FNS, 2008c), hereafter called the 2008 Diet Quality Report, and (2) the third School Nutrition Dietary Assessment study (SNDA-III) (USDA/FNS, 2007a). Both studies present data from nationally representative samples.

The committee recognizes the imprecise nature of dietary intake data and notes that the available data do not take into account contributions from dietary supplements. Because such data may not be reflective of the nutritional status of individuals (IOM, 2008), the committee views the findings as general information about food group and nutrient intakes that are likely to be of concern rather than as strong evidence of definitive problems. When terms such as "the prevalence of inadequacy" are used in reference to reported dietary intakes, the qualifiers "apparent" or "estimated" usually have been omitted for ease of reading. To broaden its perspective on schoolchildren's diets, the committee also considered selected aspects of health as related to dietary intake.

FOOD GROUP INTAKES

Assessment Method

To assess the food group intakes of schoolchildren, the committee relied on information based on the MyPyramid food guidance system (USDA, 2008). MyPyramid provides specific food-based dietary guidance that is consistent with the recommendations in the 2005 *Dietary Guidelines for Americans*. It does this by specifying food patterns for 12 calorie levels that range from 1,000 to 3,200 calories per day. To evaluate how well school-aged children's food group intakes followed *Dietary Guidelines for Americans*, the committee compared the children's mean food group intakes for one day with MyPyramid food patterns for three calorie levels as follows:

- 1,600 calories for children ages 5–8 years,
- 2,000 calories for children ages 9–13 years, and
- 2,400 calories for youth ages 14–18 years.

The committee recognizes two important limitations of these data:

1. The calorie levels and age ranges do not exactly match those determined by the committee to be most suitable for developing the Nutrient Targets and Meal Requirements. Because the committee was unable to obtain food group intake data for the 1,800 calorie level (the level selected for children ages 5 through 10 years), it used the data for the 1,600 calorie level from the 2008 Diet Quality Report instead.

2. The data had been collected 8 to 10 years ago (in the National Health and Nutrition Examination Survey 1999–2002).

Nonetheless, they were judged to be the most useful available data on food group intakes by schoolchildren. Findings from less representative studies (e.g., Kranz et al., 2009) and from SNDA-III (USDA/FNS, 2007a) are consistent with findings that appear below.[1]

Results and Discussion

Food Group Intakes

Figure 3-1 illustrates a number of useful findings about school-aged children's mean daily food group intake. Table 3-1 provides more specific information, including data on the intake of vegetable oils and discretionary calories.

As shown in Figure 3-1 and Table 3-1:

- Intake of dark green and orange vegetables, and legumes was very low (less than 20 percent of the MyPyramid amount). Whole grain consumption also was very low. Children in the youngest age group consumed only 24 percent of the MyPyramid whole grain amount, and the older children consumed even smaller percentages of the whole grain amount. *Dietary Guidelines for Americans* (HHS/USDA, 2005) specifically encourages the intake of a variety of vegetables and three or more ounce-equivalents (or at least half of the grains consumed) as whole grains each day.
- Total vegetable intake was only about 40 percent of the MyPyramid amount for the children in all three age groups. Data on the percentage of MyPyramid intakes contributed by different food sources indicate that about 29 percent of children's total vegetable intake came from potatoes (about 22 percent of the total in the form of fried potatoes or chips) (USDA/FNS, 2008c, Table C-22). The other most common food sources of vegetables were salad (greens), pizza, Italian-style pasta dishes, cooked corn, and sandwiches (excluding burgers).
- Total fruit intake was about 80 percent of the MyPyramid amount for the youngest children, which was nearly twice as high as the percentages for the older two groups of children. *Dietary Guidelines for Americans*

[1]In addition, analysis of trends in average daily per capita servings (as defined by the 2005 *Dietary Guidelines for Americans* and the MyPyramid Plan) using U.S. food availability data (adjusted for spoilage and other waste) indicates that the consumption of fruits, vegetables, and flour and cereal products has increased only between 1 and 3 percent from 2002 to 2007; but the consumption of meat, eggs, and nuts has remained constant. Data are not available to indicate the extent to which these trends hold for children (USDA/ERS, 2009).

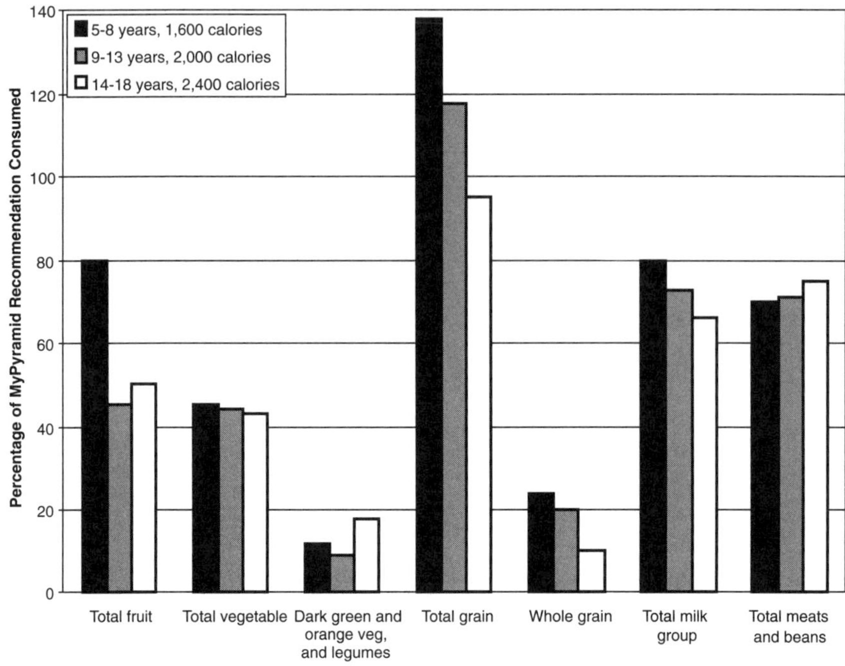

FIGURE 3-1 Percentages of MyPyramid recommendations consumed, by age group, based on the recommended daily amounts of food groups for the specified level of calories. This figure uses 3 cups rather than 2 cups as the MyPyramid recommendation for milk for the 1,600 calorie level.
NOTES: veg = vegetables. See Appendix Table H-1 for a list of foods in the MyPyramid food groups and subgroups.
SOURCE: USDA/FNS, 2008c.

recommends intake of a variety of fruits each day and a majority of the fruit intake from whole fruit rather than juice. About 78 percent of the MyPyramid fruits were contributed by a few sources: citrus juice, noncitrus juice, fresh apple, noncarbonated sweetened drink, fresh banana, fresh orange, and fresh watermelon (USDA/FNS, 2008c, Table C-21). Juice accounted for 53 percent of the MyPyramid fruit.

- Total grain intake was close to or exceeded MyPyramid amounts for all the age groups. Most of the grain products were refined. The food sources that contributed the highest percentages of the grain servings were sandwiches and burgers, pizza, cold cereal, bread, corn-based salty snacks, cookies, popcorn, and pasta dishes (USDA/FNS, 2008c, Table C-23).

TABLE 3-1 Comparison of MyPyramid Food Group Patterns with Mean Daily Amounts of MyPyramid Food Groups Consumed by Children, by Age Group

Food Group or Component[a]	1,600 kcal Pattern (5–8 y)	Mean Intake 5–8 y (n = 578)	2,000 kcal Pattern (9–13 y)	Mean Intake 9–13 y (n = 998)	2,400 kcal Pattern (14–18 y)	Mean Intake 14–18 y (n = 1,021[b])
Total fruit (cup equiv)	1.5	1.2	2.0	0.9	2.0	1.0
Total vegetables (cup equiv)	2.0	0.9	2.5	1.1	3.0	1.3
Dark green and orange vegetables and legumes	0.86[c]	0.1	1.14[c]	0.1	1.14[c]	0.2
Total grains (oz equiv)	5.0	6.9	6.0	7.1	8.0	7.6
Whole grains (oz equiv)	2.5[d]	0.6	3.0[d]	0.6	4.0[d]	0.4
Total milk group (8 fluid oz equiv)	2.0	2.4	3.0	2.2	3.0	2.0
Total meats and beans (oz equiv)	5.0	3.5	5.5	3.9	6.5	4.9
Vegetable oils (g)	22.0	14.1	27.0	15.4	31.0	18.5
Discretionary calories (kcal)	132	719[e]	267	810[e]	362	946[e]

NOTES: Weekday food consumption recalls were obtained during periods when school was in session. Estimates are based on a single 24-hour recall per child. The MyPyramid food intake pattern used is from the *Dietary Guidelines for Americans* (HHS/USDA, 2005). equiv = equivalent; g = gram; kcal = calories; oz = ounce; y = years.

[a]See Appendix Table H-1 for a list of foods in the MyPyramid food groups and subgroups.

[b]Excludes pregnant and breastfeeding females.

[c]Based on the recommendation expressed as cup equivalents per week.

[d]Based on the recommendation that half of all grain equivalents be whole grains.

[e]Estimated on the basis of the number of grams of discretionary solid fat and the number of teaspoons (tsp) of added sugars, as follows: (fat g × 9 calories/g) + (tsp × 4.2 g/tsp × 4 calories/g).

SOURCE: Weighted tabulations of data from NHANES 1999–2002, as reported in *Diet Quality of American School-Age Children by School Lunch Participation Status* (USDA/FNS, 2008c); adapted from Table C-20.

- Total milk group intake by the youngest age group exceeded the recommended intake shown in Table 3-1, but the percentage decreased with age. Data on the percentage of MyPyramid intakes contributed by different food sources indicate that about 17 percent of the total milk intake was from unflavored 2 percent milk, 16 percent from unflavored whole milk, and 9 percent from flavored milk (USDA/FNS, 2008c, Table C-24). Smaller percentages came from other sources, including cheese (either plain or in foods such as sandwiches), and unflavored low-fat and skim (fat-free) milk. A majority of the milk products consumed contained 2 percent or more milk fat, whereas *Dietary Guidelines* advises "3 cups per day of fat-free or low-fat milk or equivalent milk products"[2] for children ages 9 years and older; 2 cups per day for younger children (HHS/USDA, 2005, p. viii).
- For all three age groups, meat and bean intakes were about 70 to 75 percent of MyPyramid amounts. The food sources that were the biggest contributors to the total meat and bean intakes were sandwiches and burgers (about 31 percent combined), chicken (17 percent), beef (9 percent), and pork (4 percent).
- For all three age groups, intake of vegetable oils was about 60 percent of MyPyramid amounts. The food sources of the oils appear to be mainly fried foods, various chips, and salad dressing on different foods (USDA/FNS, 2008c, Table C-26).

Discretionary Calorie Intake

Mean daily intakes of discretionary calories from solid fats and sugars were much higher than the amounts specified by MyPyramid for the three age groups. Based on calculations shown in the Phase I report (IOM, 2008, Table 4-5) and summarized in Table 3-1 above, children ages 5–8 years consumed, on average, 587 calories more from solid fats and added sugars than were in the MyPyramid plan. The discretionary calorie excesses were somewhat lower for the older age groups: 543 calories for children ages 9–13 years and 584 calories for children ages 14–18 years. Clearly, children's intakes of solid fats and added sugars were undesirably high when compared with recommendations in *Dietary Guidelines for Americans* (HHS/USDA, 2005). Many food sources contributed discretionary solid fat. The highest contributor was sandwiches including burgers (15 percent) (USDA/FNS, 2008c, Table C-27). The next highest contributors were fried potatoes and pizza with meat, which contributed about 6 percent each. By far the largest contributors to the intakes of added sugars (45 percent of the total amount) were regular soda and noncarbonated sweetened drinks.

---

[2]Low-fat milk is defined as having 1 percent milk fat.

Summary of Food Group Intakes

Overall, these data indicate that dietary changes to improve consistency with *Dietary Guidelines for Americans* would feature increased intake of a variety of vegetables, whole fruits, and whole grains; increased emphasis on low-fat or fat-free milk products; increased emphasis on very lean meats and/or beans; and decreased intake of foods high in solid fat, added sugars, or both.

ENERGY AND NUTRIENT INTAKES

As stated in *Dietary Reference Intakes: Applications in Dietary Planning*:

> Dietary planning and assessment are inextricably linked.
>
> (IOM, 2003, p. 27)

Thus, an early step in the committee's planning process was the assessment of schoolchildren's estimated dietary intake of energy and nutrients.

The Dietary Reference Intakes (DRIs) provided the reference values used for the dietary intake assessment. DRIs are nutrient reference values developed for the United States and Canada for use in the assessment and planning of diets for healthy people. A complete set of the values appears in *Dietary Reference Intakes: The Essential Guide to Nutrient Requirements* (IOM, 2006). The DRIs comprise five types of reference values: the Estimated Average Requirement (EAR), Adequate Intake (AI), Recommended Dietary Allowance (RDA), Tolerable Upper Intake Level (UL), and Acceptable Macronutrient Distribution Range (AMDR). Box 3-1 provides definitions for the DRIs that are used to plan and assess group intakes.

To assess intakes, the committee used methods recommended and described by the Institute of Medicine for the assessment of energy and nutrient intakes (IOM, 2000b). These methods make use of the EAR, the AI, and the UL, but not the RDA. The Estimated Energy Requirement, a calculated value, is used in assessing energy intakes. The methods used in applying the different types of reference values are described in the following sections.

SNDA-III (USDA/FNS, 2007a) provided 24-hour dietary intake data on schoolchildren's intakes of energy and nutrients but no data on intakes from dietary supplements. The assessments were conducted for the age-grade groups identified in Chapter 3: 6–10 years,[3] 11–13 years, and 14–18 years.

---

[3]Because SNDA-III did not collect data on children 5 years of age, this age group spans fewer years that the one specified by the committee.

BOX 3-1
Definitions of Dietary Reference Intakes Used to Plan and Assess Group Intakes

Estimated Average Requirement (EAR): Level of nutrient in a diet that meets the needs of 50 percent of a population. The EAR may be used as a cut-point to estimate the prevalence of inadequate intakes in a group.

Adequate Intake (AI): An AI has been set for some nutrients, rather than an EAR. The AI is interpreted as the median intake of a healthy population, although the methods for setting AIs have varied. The AI may be used as the goal for the median intake of a population, although the actual prevalence of inadequacy cannot be estimated.

Tolerable Upper Intake Level (UL): The level of intake of a nutrient that is associated with little or no risk of having adverse effects. For a population group, the proportion of usual intakes above the UL is interpreted as the prevalence of excessive intakes.

Some of the nutrient intake values and other nutrient findings presented in this report differ from those in the Phase I report (IOM, 2008) for the younger two age-grade groups because of differences in the age spans used. New analyses were conducted to examine, by gender, the intakes of schoolchildren in each age-grade group.

Energy

The committee used the SNDA-III data to estimate mean and median energy intake as well as energy expenditure for the children by age-grade group and gender. Energy expenditure was estimated for comparison with reported intake. Each child's age, weight, and height were entered in the DRI equations (IOM, 2002/2005) for calculating the Estimated Energy Requirement. Because data on physical activity were not collected in SNDA-III, the physical activity level assumptions shown in Table 2-3 in Chapter 2 were used to select the physical activity coefficient in the equations. The mean Estimated Energy Requirement was then calculated for all children in each age-grade-gender group.

Major discrepancies were found between the mean energy intake that was estimated using the SNDA-III data and the mean Estimated Energy Requirement that was calculated as described in Chapter 2. For example, reported usual energy intakes exceeded the mean Estimated Energy Requirement by about 400 calories for the younger children and the energy intakes were lower than the Estimated Energy Requirement for the adolescents ages 14–18 years. These discrepancies were not unexpected, considering the potential for (1) overreporting total food intake of the younger children and underestimating their physical activity level and (2) underreporting total food intake of the adolescents and overestimating their physical activity level. With regard to physical activity level, SNDA-III assumed a low-active level regardless of age. Although these discrepancies limited the committee's ability to draw conclusions about the adequacy of energy intake using survey data, data on the prevalence of childhood overweight and obesity provide strong reason for concern about excessive calorie intake (see "Obesity" under "Supportive Findings" in this chapter).

Nutrients with an Estimated Average Requirement

For nutrients that have an EAR, the assessment of intake entails analysis to obtain the prevalence of inadequacy. The committee examined the distribution of usual intake of the 14 nutrients for which the DRI value is an EAR and estimated the prevalence of inadequacy of each by age-grade group and gender. It used the EAR cut-point method (IOM, 2001) for the estimations for all nutrients except iron for the older females. That is, for females ages 11–13 years and 14–18 years, the committee used the probability approach (IOM, 2000b, pp. 205–208) to estimate the prevalence of inadequate iron intake (see Appendix Tables I-2 and I-3 and also "Supportive Findings" in this chapter). Appendix Table I-1 presents data to allow comparison of the EAR for 14 nutrients with the reported usual intakes of those nutrients at the 5th percentile and at the median (50th percentile).

For most of the nutrients, based on the SNDA-III data, the 5th percentile of intake equals or exceeds the EAR, implying a low prevalence of inadequacy. The most obvious exception is vitamin E—even the median intake was below the EAR for all age and gender groups, meaning that the prevalence of inadequacy exceeds 50 percent. The estimated prevalence of usual intakes at or below the EAR is less than 3 percent for many nutrients (the B vitamins especially) (see Table 3-2). Notable exceptions (that is, nutrients with relatively high prevalence of inadequacy) include vitamin A, vitamin E, magnesium, and phosphorus. The estimated prevalence of inadequacy of vitamin E exceeded 80 percent for all age-gender groups. For 14–18-year-old females, the prevalence of inadequacy ranged from 7 to 97 percent across all the nutrients, and it was especially high for vitamins A, C, and E; folate; magnesium; phosphorus; and zinc. The prevalence of inadequacy also tended to be high for females ages 11–13 years, but to a lesser degree. The findings for the older adolescent females are consistent with their very low reported mean energy intakes.

TABLE 3-2 Estimated Prevalence of Inadequacy of Protein and Selected Vitamins and Minerals Among Schoolchildren Based on Usual Nutrient Intakes from SNDA-III[a]

	Estimated Prevalence of Inadequate Usual Intakes (%)					
	6–10 years		11–13 years		14–18 years	
Nutrient	Males (n = 295)	Females (n = 317)	Males (n = 342)	Females (n = 342)	Males (n = 506)	Females (n = 512)
Protein[b]	< 3[c]	< 3	< 3	**9**	< 3	**16**
Vitamin A	**6**	**6**	**11**	**30**	**49**	**58**
Vitamin C	**6**	< 3	3	**16**	**27**	**40**
Vitamin E	**84**	**81**	**87**	**87**	**95**	> **97**[d]
Thiamin	< 3	< 3	< 3	4	3*	**17**
Riboflavin	< 3	< 3	< 3	< 3	< 3	**7***
Niacin	< 3	< 3	< 3	< 3	< 3	**9***
Vitamin B_6	< 3	< 3	< 3	5	< 3	**20**
Folate	< 3	< 3	< 3	7	< 3	**24**
Vitamin B_{12}	< 3	< 3	< 3	< 3	< 3	**13***
Phosphorus	**6**	**6**	4	**38**	**9***	**46**
Magnesium	5	**8**	**11**	**35**	**72**	**87**
Iron	< 3	< 3	< 3	**11**[e]	< 3	**15**[e]
Zinc	< 3	4	< 3	**13**	**7***	**28**

NOTES: n = sample size; SNDA-III = third School Nutrition Dietary Assessment study; y = years; *point estimate may not be reliable because of inadequate cell size or a large coefficient of variation. Bold font indicates values with a prevalence of inadequacy greater than 5 percent.

[a]All nutrients in this table have an Estimated Average Requirement (EAR).

[b]The sample sizes for protein data, which are smaller than those for the other nutrients, are as follows: males 6–10 years, 284; females 6–10 years, 306; males 11–13 years, 334; females 11–13 years, 328; males 14–18 years, 494; females 14–18 years, 482.

[c]Less than 3 percent is reported when less than 3 percent of students had usual intakes in this range, but the specific point estimate was statistically unreliable.

[d]More than 97 percent is reported for common occurrences (more than 97 percent of students have usual intakes in this range, but the specific point estimate was statistically unreliable).

[e]Calculated using the probability approach and, for the 11–13-year-old females, an adjusted EAR value. See Appendix I and also "Iron Status" under "Supportive Findings" in this chapter.

SOURCES: Weighted tabulations of data from SNDA-III (USDA/FNS, 2007a); Dietary intake data (24-hour recalls) were collected during the 2004–2005 school year and do not include intakes from dietary supplements (e.g., multivitamin-multimineral preparations). The personal computer version of the Software for Intake Distribution Estimation (PC-SIDE; ISU, 1997) was used to estimate the usual nutrient intake distributions and the percentage of children with usual intakes below the EAR. The EARs used in the analysis were from the Dietary Reference Intake reports (IOM, 1997, 1998, 2000a, 2001, 2002/2005).

Nutrients with an Adequate Intake

The committee examined the distribution of intake for five nutrients with an AI, but it focused on mean intake. This approach was used because the prevalence of inadequate usual intakes cannot be estimated for nutrients that have an AI rather than an EAR (IOM, 2000b). Groups with mean intakes at or above the AI, however, can generally be assumed to have a low prevalence of inadequacy. Assumptions about the prevalence of inadequacy of intakes cannot be made when the mean intake is below the AI.

Sodium, another nutrient with an AI, is not included in Table 3-3 and is discussed separately, relative to the UL, because the concern is for excessive rather than inadequate sodium intake. Because SNDA-III provided no data on vitamin D intake and no other reliable data sources provided the type of data needed, the committee did not assess vitamin D intake. The very recent What We Eat in America (NHANES 2005–2006) survey (USDA/ARS, 2009a) includes estimates of vitamin D intakes (for different age groups than those used by the committee) and shows low intakes, especially for adolescent females.

Table 3-3 shows that mean intakes of potassium and fiber were below the AI for all three age-grade groups and that mean intake of calcium was below the AI for the older two age-grade groups. The mean intakes of linoleic and α-linolenic acids were above the AI for all three age-grade groups.

It is important to note that another committee of the Institute of Medicine is conducting a study to assess current relevant data on vitamin D and calcium and, if appropriate, to update the DRIs for those two nutrients. It is possible that the committee's findings will have implications for the assessment of schoolchildren's intakes of these two nutrients.

Nutrients with a Tolerable Upper Intake Level

Because no data sources available to the committee provided information about contributions to nutrient intake from supplements, the committee's assessment of usual nutrient intakes relative to the UL was limited. Eight of the nutrients considered by the committee have ULs. The committee compared the usual nutrient intake distributions of four of these—calcium, iron, phosphorus, and zinc—with the defined ULs for the age-grade groups. The other four were considered differently, as described below. For males and females within each age-grade group, intakes at the 95th percentile of the distribution were well below the ULs for all but zinc. More than 17 percent of children ages 6–10 years had usual zinc intakes that exceeded their UL. Intakes that exceeded the UL were seen mainly among the 6–8-year-old children in this 6–10-year-old group. For the younger children, the

TABLE 3-3 Comparison of Mean Nutrient Intakes with the Adequate Intake (AI), by Age-Grade Group and Gender

Nutrient	6–10 years		11–13 years		14–18 years	
	Males (n = 295)	Females (n = 317)	Males (n = 342)	Females (n = 342)	Males (n = 506)	Females (n = 512)
Calcium (mg/d)						
AI	1,000	1,000	1,300	1,300	1,300	1,300
Mean intake	1,176	1,086	**1,237**	**949**	**1,248**	**847**
Potassium (mg/d)						
AI	4,080	4,080	4,500	4,500	4,700	4,700
Mean intake	**2,562**	**2,379**	**2,700**	**2,289**	**3,005**	**2,081**
Fiber (g/d)						
AI	27.4	25.4	31.0	26.0	38.0	26.0
Mean intake	**14.6**	**13.6**	**15.1**	**12.8**	**16.2**	**12.0**
Linoleic acid (g/d)						
AI	10.8	10.0	12.0	10.0	16.0	11.0
Mean intake	13.1	11.6	14.2	12.7	16.5	12.0
α-Linolenic acid (g/d)						
AI	1.0	0.9	1.2	1.0	1.6	1.1
Mean intake	1.2	1.1	1.3	1.2	1.6	1.2

NOTES: AI = Adequate Intake; g/d = grams per day; mg/d = milligrams per day; n = sample size. Bold font indicates mean intake values lower than the AI.
SOURCES: Weighted tabulations of data from SNDA-III (USDA/FNS, 2007a). The AIs used in the analysis were from the DRI reports (IOM, 1997, 2002/2005, 2005). AIs shown for the males and females ages 6–10 years are weighted averages of two DRI age groups.

UL is 12 mg and their intake at the 75th percentile of the distribution was 12.6 mg (Zlotkin, 2006). For older children, whose UL is much higher, zinc intakes at the 95th percentile of the distribution were well below the UL.

Intakes of folate, niacin, and magnesium appear to exceed the UL for at least some age-gender groups, but the assessment needs to consider the form of the nutrient used in setting the UL. Because the ULs for magnesium represent intake from a pharmacological agent only, they do not apply to dietary intake. The ULs for folate and niacin apply only to the synthetic forms of these vitamins (the forms that are present in certain fortified and enriched foods). Lack of data on the content of the synthetic forms of the vitamins in foods limits the ability to assess the potential for excessive intake of folate and niacin.

Sodium intake clearly was excessive. The SNDA-III study (USDA/FNS, 2007a) found that mean daily sodium intake for all schoolchildren ages 6–18 years was 3,404 mg, and intake at the 95th percentile was 5,270 mg. These values contrast sharply with the ULs for sodium, which are 1,900 mg for children ages 4–8 years, 2,200 mg for those 11–13 years, and 2,300 mg for children ages 14–18 years. Overall, more than 90 percent of schoolchildren had usual sodium intake that exceeded the UL.

Fats and Cholesterol

Dietary Guidelines for Americans (HHS/USDA, 2005) provides recommendations for total fat, saturated fat, and cholesterol; but DRIs have been established only for total fat (IOM, 2002/2005).[4] Therefore, the committee used the *Dietary Guidelines* recommendations in assessing schoolchildren's intakes of saturated fat, total fat, and cholesterol. Both the 2008 Diet Quality Report and the SNDA-III provide data on the proportions of children whose usual intakes of saturated fat, total fat, and cholesterol exceeded the maximum intakes recommended and on the proportions of children whose usual intakes of total fat were below the recommended minimum. The values cited below are based on SNDA-III data. Although *Dietary Guidelines* recommends that intake of *trans* fat be as low as possible, no reliable data were available for use in assessing schoolchildren's intake of that food component. For further discussion of *trans* fats, see Chapter 4.

Saturated Fat

Dietary Guidelines for Americans (HHS/USDA, 2005) specifies that less than 10 percent of total food energy should be provided by saturated fat (regardless of age or gender). Because this recommendation is based on calorie intake, the number of grams of saturated fat set as the maximum differs by age and gender. It is considerably higher for active adolescent males than for sedentary adolescent females, for example. Nearly 80 percent of children in all the age-gender subgroups had usual saturated fat intakes that exceeded the recommended limit.

Total Fat

For school-aged children, *Dietary Guidelines for Americans* gives a range of 25 to 35 percent of calories for total fat intake, not just a maximum. More than 75 percent of children in all age-grade groups had usual fat intakes that were within this range. About 19 percent of all children had total fat intake that was above 35 percent of calories. Less than 3 percent of schoolchildren had reported usual fat intakes that were below 25 percent

[4]The recommendations on total fat intake in *Dietary Guidelines* are the same as the Acceptable Macronutrient Distribution Range (AMDR) for fat—the type of DRI that is used for fat.

of calories except for females ages 14–18 years (about 9 percent of these adolescents had low reported fat intakes) (USDA/FNS, 2008c).

Cholesterol

Dietary Guidelines recommends 300 mg of cholesterol as the maximum daily intake (for all persons who are at least 2 years of age). Cholesterol intakes were fairly consistent with the recommendation: more than 85 percent of all schoolchildren had usual cholesterol intakes that were not more than 300 mg per day. The prevalence of excessive cholesterol intakes was higher for males than for females and was highest among adolescent males (nearly 20 percent for males ages 11–13 years and nearly 37 percent for males ages 14–18 years), partially reflecting the fact that the recommendation is the same regardless of calorie needs.

Considerations Regarding the Identification of Priority Nutrients

The committee examined its findings on nutrient intakes to determine whether it would be appropriate to focus on a subset of the nutrients in setting Nutrient Targets or Meal Requirements, or both. A subset called *key nutrients* (calories, protein, vitamins A and C, calcium, iron, total fat, and saturated fat) had been used in developing the existing Nutrition Standards for school meals. A different subset of five *nutrients of concern* (calcium, potassium, fiber, magnesium, and vitamin E) is identified for children and adolescents in *Dietary Guidelines for Americans* (HHS/USDA, 2005). *Dietary Guidelines* also focuses on saturated fat, total fat, *trans* fat, cholesterol, and sodium. The report *Healthy People 2010 Objectives for the Nation* (HHS, 2000) lists public health objectives for saturated fat, total fat, calcium, and sodium but no other nutrients.

The committee's assessment of schoolchildren's dietary intakes of a set of 23 nutrients[5] suggests low intakes of the same nutrients of concern as identified by *Dietary Guidelines*, but the assessment also points to a relatively high prevalence of inadequacy of vitamin A, vitamin C, and phosphorus for several of the age-grade groups and of most vitamins and minerals for females ages 14–18 years—all of which might be called nutrients of concern or *shortfall nutrients* at least for some age-grade groups. Sodium intake was excessive for all age-grade groups, and saturated fat intake was excessive for more than 75 percent of the children.

The committee searched the literature but found no convincing evidence that achieving adequate intakes of a small number of nutrients could serve as a valid proxy for achieving adequate intakes of all the nutrients. More-

[5]This statement excludes calories.

over, nutrition labeling information is not required for four of the nutrients (potassium, magnesium, vitamin E, and phosphorus) that could be termed shortfall nutrients for at least several age-grade groups. Thus, although subsets of nutrients are useful for various public health purposes, the committee determined that it is valuable to use a more complete set of nutrients when developing Nutrient Targets in the design of the Meal Requirements for school meals. This approach avoids the possibility that a nutrient such as potassium, for example, will be overlooked in developing standards for menu planning. Therefore, the committee considered all 23 nutrients as it developed its method for setting standards for menu planning. The methods used to set targets for the nutrients appear in Chapter 4.

SUPPORTIVE FINDINGS

To complete its assessment of schoolchildren's food and nutrient intakes, the committee searched for recent physical data that would support the dietary findings. In addition, recent Institute of Medicine reports (IOM, 2007a, 2007b) and targeted literature searches covering the past few years provided a useful perspective on associations of children's health with weight status and with selected aspects of diet. This section briefly covers overweight and obesity, blood pressure, calcium and vitamin D, iron status, and folate status. The information points to the key role that an appropriate calorie intake and a nutritious diet have in the prevention of many chronic conditions.

Obesity[6]

The committee turned to physical evidence on weight status and studies of associations of weight status with health to gain perspective on the importance of setting appropriate calorie levels for school meals.

Defining Overweight and Obesity in Children

The terms overweight and obesity are meant to reflect an amount of body fat that is elevated to a level that has clear adverse effects on health. The definitions for overweight and obesity are based on the body mass index (BMI), which is calculated as the weight in kilograms divided by height in meters squared: kg/m^2. This index is an expression of body weight (mass) adjusted for height, and it is a good proxy for body fatness at the *popula-*

[6]Some of the content in this section is derived from the report *Nutrition Standards for School Foods: Leading the Way Toward Healthier Youth* (IOM, 2007a), with recent updates, and from the Phase I report (IOM, 2008).

tion level. This report uses the age- and gender-specific reference data for BMI for children published by the Centers for Disease Control and Prevention (Kuczmarski et al., 2000). Children and adolescents with a BMI over the 95th percentile are termed *obese* and those between the 85th and 95th percentiles *overweight* (CDC, 2009).

Prevalence of Obesity Among U.S. Schoolchildren Has Increased

Much concern has been raised about the increasing prevalence of obesity among U.S. children, as indicated by the age- and gender-specific BMIs at the 95th percentile or higher (CDC, 2008). From 1976 to 2006, striking increases in the percentages of obese children occurred, as shown in Figure 3-2.

Table 3-4 presents recent data on three categories of high BMIs among U.S. children. Notably, nearly one-third of all children are overweight or obese (BMI ≥ 85th percentile). Specifically, close to 17 percent of children are obese (BMI > 95th percentile for age and gender) and 16 percent are overweight. For each age group, the prevalence of obesity and of overweight are higher among males than among females and higher among non-Hispanic blacks and Mexican Americans than among non-Hispanic whites (data not shown) (Ogden et al., 2008).

Health Risks for Children: Obesity Matters

Despite the limitations in the use of BMI as a measure of pediatric obesity (Ebbeling and Ludwig, 2008), the prevalences of obesity shown in Table 3-4 indicate that large numbers of children and adolescents are at increased risk for chronic disease: type II diabetes (Messiah et al., 2008; Weiss and Caprio, 2005), hypertension (Jago et al., 2006), and metabolic syndrome (De Ferranti et al., 2006) in the short term and both diabetes and cardiovascular disease in the long term (Baker et al., 2007). In addition, children who are overweight are at increased risk of becoming overweight adults, with all the attendant risks and compromises to good health that are implied (Ferraro et al., 2003). Moreover, overweight children may experience social stigma and emotional ill health (Anderson et al., 2006; French et al., 1995). In a recent multisite, multiethnic study of adolescents, Wallander et al. (2009) found that psychosocial quality-of-life (but not physical quality-of-life) measures were lower for obese than for nonobese children. A recent Arkansas study documented poorer academic performance among overweight children, mediated largely through weight-related teasing by peers (Krukowski et al., 2009).

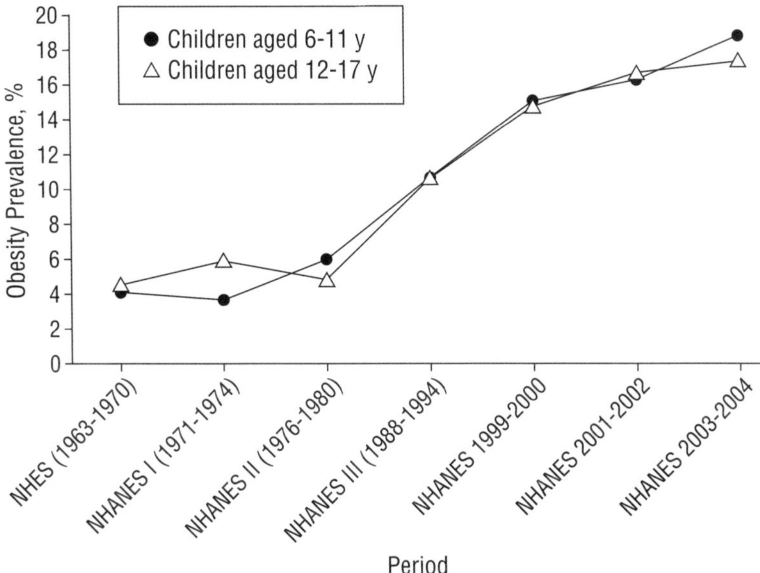

FIGURE 3-2 Trends in obesity prevalence among U.S. children.
NOTES: NHANES = National Health and Nutrition Examination Survey; NHES = National Health Examination Survey; y = years.
SOURCE: Lee, 2008. Reprinted with permission from Archives of Pediatrics and Adolescent Medicine. July 2008. 162(7):683. Copyright © American Medical Association. All rights reserved.

Role of School Breakfast and Lunch Programs in Relation to Childhood Obesity

No definitive studies have been found that provide evidence of how the school meal programs affect children's weight status. However, a recent analysis of data from SNDA-III indicated that School Breakfast Program participants had significantly lower BMI than did nonparticipants and that there were racial/ethnic differences in the associations of BMI with participation (Gleason and Dodd, 2009). Because of the substantial contribution of school meals to many children's total calorie and nutrient intake during the school years, revision of the current Nutrition Standards and Meal Requirements might hold potential for reducing any possible contribution of the school meal programs to childhood obesity. The amount of time that children spend at school and the substantial proportion of their dietary intake that can be derived from school meals dictates that school meals be structured in such a way that they do not contribute to childhood obe-

TABLE 3-4 Prevalence of High BMIs Among U.S. Children, by Age, 2003–2006

Age Group (in years, both genders)	Percentage of Children (SE) with the Following BMIs According to CDC Growth Charts		
	≥ 97th Percentile	≥ 95th Percentile	≥ 85th Percentile
6–11	11.4 (0.9)	17.0 (1.3)	33.3 (2.0)
12–19	12.6 (1.0)	17.6 (1.2)	34.1 (1.5)

NOTES: Data come from the National Health and Nutrition Examination Survey. Pregnant adolescents were excluded. Values for BMIs were rounded to one decimal place. CDC = Centers for Disease Control and Prevention; SE = standard error.
SOURCE: Derived from Ogden et al., 2008. Reprinted with permission from Journal of the American Medicine Association. May 28, 2008. 299(20):2403. Copyright © American Medical Association. All rights reserved.

sity. On the other hand, neither school meals nor the school environment provide appropriate venues for the treatment or clinical management of overweight and obesity among schoolchildren. Because of concerns about children from households with low food security coupled with concerns about childhood obesity, the calorie levels for school meals need to be high enough to meet the needs of the students on average.

Blood Pressure

Using data on children from the third National Health and Nutrition Examination Survey (NHANES III, 1988–1994) and from NHANES 1999–2000, Muntner and colleagues (2004) provided evidence that part of the observed increase in blood pressure over the past decade is attributable to the increase in prevalence of overweight that occurred over the same period. Sodium intake also appears to be related to children's blood pressure, and high blood pressure responds to a reduction in salt intake in children as in adults (He and MacGregor, 2006; Pappadis and Somers, 2003). A recent, large cross-sectional population study of adolescents in the United Kingdom shows a clear relationship between blood pressure and salt intake, independent of BMI (He et al., 2008). Such studies provide support for efforts to support healthy weight among children and to reduce their intakes of sodium.

Calcium and Vitamin D

Late childhood and the adolescent years provide the window of opportunity to influence lifelong bone health. Approximately 45 percent of the adult skeleton is acquired between the ages of 9 and 17 years (Weaver and Heaney, 2006). Because the amount of bone accumulated during pubertal growth depends to some extent on the amount of calcium and vitamin D in the diet, an adequate intake of these nutrients during childhood and adolescence is critical to bone health (Greer et al., 2006; Heaney et al., 2000).

Recently, considerable attention has been focused on the requirements for vitamin D, the vitamin D status of the U.S. population, and the potential roles of vitamin D in health. The related discussions and controversies include questions regarding the adequate intake of vitamin D among schoolchildren. Such questions remain unresolved, however. Recently, an Institute of Medicine committee was convened to review available data and, if appropriate, revise the DRIs for vitamin D. Calcium also was included in this study. The report on this activity is scheduled for release in mid-2010. Until the important work of the DRI committee is completed, it would be premature to make conclusions about vitamin D concerns as they may relate to schoolchildren. The topic, however, is relevant to the goals of this committee's work because school meals may play an important role in helping schoolchildren consume adequate amounts of calcium and vitamin D. Thus, any relevant recommendations from the upcoming Institute of Medicine report should be taken into account by those responsible for ensuring that school meals address children's nutritional needs.

Iron Status

Laboratory data are available on which to base reliable estimates of iron deficiency. According to NHANES 1999–2000 data (CDC, 2002) for children ages 6–11 years, 4 percent had iron deficiency, defined as having an abnormal value for at least two of the following: serum ferritin, transferrin saturation, and erythrocyte protoporphyrin.[7] The prevalence of iron deficiency was 9 percent among females ages 12–15 years, 16 percent among females ages 16–19 years, and lower for the other age-gender groups.

The relatively high prevalence of iron deficiency among adolescent females and the known adverse effects of iron deficiency and anemia led the committee to consider the value to use for the Estimated Average Requirement (EAR) for females ages 11–13 years. The physiological changes that occur during adolescence complicate the setting of the EAR for iron (IOM, 2001), especially for the DRI age range of 9–13 years. The current EAR for girls 9–13 years assumes that girls in this age range do not menstruate. However, the average age of menarche in the United States is about

[7]Cutpoints by age were as follows: for serum ferritin, 6+ years, < 12 μg/L. For transferrin saturation, 6–15 years, < 14%; 16+ years, < 15%. For erythrocyte protoporphyrin, 3+ years, > 1.24 μmol/L red blood cells (Cusick et al., 2008).

12.5 years, meaning that more than half of all girls will be menstruating by age 13 years. The accompanying median blood loss is estimated to increase the iron requirement by 0.45 mg of iron per day (IOM, 2001). For some subgroups of the population, the average age of menarche is even earlier (Chumlea et al., 2003). In addition, in girls the growth spurt that accompanies puberty usually begins before menarche. Tanner et al. (1966) showed that growth velocity peaks at 12–13 years among girls, and the growth spurt also requires additional iron (an additional 1.3 mg per day for girls) (IOM, 2001). Therefore it is reasonable to assume that a substantial number of girls ages 11–13 years will be experiencing a growth spurt and will be menstruating. On this basis, the committee concluded that an adjustment is needed for the purpose of setting the iron target for girls in the 11–13-year age-grade group. In particular, the EAR for iron (5.7 mg per day) needs to be increased by 1.8 mg per day (0.5 mg for menstruation and 1.3 mg for the growth spurt) for the middle school girls.

> Conclusion: For the purposes of setting Nutrient Targets for school meals, the value used for the EAR for iron for girls ages 11–13 years will be 7.5 mg per day. This is a conservative estimate of the mean iron requirement that will ensure that the Nutrient Target will be applicable to populations of girls who are menstruating and experiencing the adolescent growth spurt.

Folate Status

The measurement of serum folate concentrations of various subgroups confirms findings of changes in folate intake that have occurred since 1998, when the Food and Drug Administration first required the addition of folic acid (a synthetic form of folate) to enrich cereal grains and bakery products. Serum folate values increased between 119 to 161 percent during the first postfortification period (1999–2000) (Briefel and Johnson, 2004). Using the same NHANES data set, the estimated intakes of folate also increased. Although serum folate values have declined slightly from the first postfortification values, they remain well above prefortification values (Pfeiffer et al., 2007). Clearly, the fortification of enriched grain products has contributed important amounts of folate to the dietary intakes of many Americans.

SUMMARY AND CONCLUSIONS

This review of dietary intake data has identified a number of foods and nutrients for which a notable proportion of children had intake levels inconsistent with reference intake levels. All the age-grade groups had mean daily intakes of fruits, vegetables (especially dark green and orange vegetables and legumes), whole grains, total meat and beans, and milk products that were lower than MyPyramid amounts. Across the entire age range, the prevalence of inadequacy was very high for vitamin E, but no health consequences have been associated with these reported intakes of vitamin E. Mean intakes of potassium and fiber also were low. For both males and females ages 9 years and older, the prevalence of inadequate intakes of magnesium and vitamin A was high. Adolescent females tended to have low reported intakes of nearly all the nutrients investigated by the committee. This finding is consistent with the low reported energy intakes of many adolescent females.

Based on food intake data, children's mean intake of discretionary calories from solid fats and added sugars was much higher than the amounts shown by the MyPyramid food patterns. For all the age groups, nutrient analysis showed that very high percentages of the children had excessive intakes of sodium and saturated fat,[8] and high usual intake of total fat was also common.

Despite limitations of the data on energy intake and energy requirements of the schoolchildren, the finding of energy consumption that exceeds the estimated average energy requirement among the younger children is a concern in the setting of the high prevalence of childhood overweight and obesity. Overweight and obesity are of great concern because of associated health and psychosocial risks, especially if the excess weight is carried into the adult years. Reconsideration of calcium and vitamin D status and needs may be necessary pending the release of an upcoming Institute of Medicine report on these two nutrients. Recent data support the value of reducing sodium intake to help control blood pressure. Evidence is presented to explain the committee's decision to adjust the iron requirement upward for middle school females. Laboratory data indicate that the folate status of children improved after enactment of the federal requirement for the folic acid fortification of enriched grain products.

Clearly there is room for improvement of children's dietary intakes. The chapter lends support to the position that attention to nutritious meals in the school meal programs may contribute to children's current and future health and well-being.

---

[8]This is consistent with high mean intake of solid fats.

4

Process for Developing the Nutrient Targets

The committee developed Nutrient Targets to serve as a guide for setting the standards for menu planning. It did so for 24 nutrients and other dietary components. The full range of nutrients needed to be considered to be certain that the standards for menu planning would be developed appropriately. The intent is not to use the Nutrient Targets themselves for menu planning.

In developing the Nutrient Targets, the committee took several different approaches that depended on the type of nutrient. This chapter describes the approaches used to set preliminary targets for (1) calories, (2) fats and cholesterol, (3) nutrients with Estimated Average Requirements, and (4) nutrients with Adequate Intakes. The term *nutrient target* is used to denote each preliminary value. Chapter 5 covers the process for using nutrient targets in developing recommended Meal Requirements, Chapter 6 covers the iterative process that led to the final recommendations, and Chapter 7 presents the recommended Nutrient Targets and Meal Requirements.

PRELIMINARY CALORIE TARGETS FOR MEALS

Method Used to Set Calorie Targets for Breakfast and Lunch for the Three Age-Grade Groups

As described in Chapter 2, the committee set mean daily calorie levels for each of the three age-grade groups (combining means for males and females) and then rounded these values to have them correspond with My-

TABLE 4-1 Mean and Rounded MyPyramid Calorie Levels by Age-Grade Group

Age-Grade Group	Mean Calorie Level for Males and Females[a]	Rounded Calorie Level for Males and Females
Ages 5–10 y, Kindergarten–Grade 5	1,830	1,800
Ages 11–13 y, Grade 6–8	2,015	2,000
Ages 14–18 y, Grade 9–12	2,365	2,400

NOTE: y = years.

[a]These requirements were obtained from the mean Estimated Energy Requirement calculations for the age-grade-gender group.

Pyramid calorie levels for meal patterns. The original and rounded mean values appear in Table 4-1.

To determine target calorie levels for school breakfast and lunch, the committee reviewed data from the third School Nutrition Dietary Assessment study (SNDA-III). These data (shown in Appendix G, Table G-1) indicated that, compared with a single value, a range would more accurately represent the proportion of calories obtained by school-aged children from meals and snacks. The children who participated in the School Breakfast Program obtained 19 to 24 percent of their total calorie intake from breakfast. The children who participated in the National School Lunch Program obtained approximately 30 to 34 percent of their total calorie intake (over 24 hours) from lunch. Findings were comparable for school-aged children overall and for low-income children (those approved for free or reduced-price meal benefits) (data not shown). The committee also reviewed data from the National Health and Nutrition Examination Survey (NHANES) 1999–2004 and found that the distribution of calories among breakfast, lunch, dinner, and snacks was consistent with that found using SNDA-III data.

The committee agreed to set a maximum target for calories to help limit excessive calorie intake at breakfast and lunch. Having both a minimum and a maximum value helps ensure adequate calories while giving school food operators some flexibility when planning menus. The means of the values used for the minimum and maximum calories (21.5 percent for breakfast and 32 percent for lunch) were used in setting selected Nutrient Targets, as described later in this chapter.

The committee applied the information about the proportion of calories that children typically obtain from breakfast and lunch meals to the rounded calorie levels established for the three age-grade groups. For example, for children ages 5–10 years, the lower end of the calorie range was calculated as follows:

$$\text{lunch calories} = 1{,}800 \text{ calories} \times 0.3$$

To provide calorie targets that would be practical for school food operators, the committee agreed to use rounded values to establish the target calorie values for each meal. They were rounded to the nearest 50 while retaining at least a 100-calorie range within an age-grade group.

Results and Discussion

Tables 4-2 and 4-3 show the values used to set the preliminary target minimum and maximum calorie values for school breakfast and school lunch, respectively, and the rounded target calorie values. These values apply to the average daily calorie content of meals *offered* across a 5-day school week. The calorie content of the meals offered on a single day could be below the minimum or above the maximum as long as the average for the week falls within the range.

The committee recognizes that some children with limited access to food or with substantially higher calorie needs might benefit from school meals that provide significantly more calories (and nutrients). It believes, however, that this situation does not provide the basis for an increase in the

TABLE 4-2 Values Used to Set Preliminary Target Calorie Minimum and Maximum for School Breakfast and Preliminary Target Calories, by Age-Grade Group

Age-Grade Group	Mean Daily Calories	Minimum: 19% of Daily	Maximum: 24% of Daily	Preliminary Target Minimum and Maximum
Ages 5–10 y, Kindergarten–Grade 5	1,800	342	432	350–450
Ages 11–13 y, Grades 6–8	2,000	380	480	400–500
Ages 14–18 y, Grades 9–12	2,400	456	576	450–600

NOTE: y = years.

TABLE 4-3 Values Used to Set Preliminary Target Calorie Minimum and Maximum for School Lunch and Preliminary Target Calories, by Age-Grade Group

Age-Grade Group	Mean Daily Calories	Minimum: 30% of Daily	Maximum: 34% of Daily	Preliminary Target Minimum and Maximum
Ages 5–10 y, Kindergarten–Grade 5	1,800	540	612	550–650
Ages 11–13 y, Grades 6–8	2,000	600	680	600–700
Ages 14–18 y, Grades 9–12	2,400	720	816	700–800

NOTE: y = years.

maximum calorie levels for school meals. Instead, school food authorities and community organizations have additional mechanisms to help ensure that children have access to sufficient food during the day.

SETTING THE MAXIMUM FOR SATURATED FAT AND CHOLESTEROL, THE RANGES FOR TOTAL FAT, AND ADDRESSING *TRANS* FAT

The committee relied on recommendations from *Dietary Guidelines for Americans* to set a target *maximum* intake for saturated fat and cholesterol (substances in food that are not essential nutrients) and the range for total fat. It considered *Dietary Guidelines* plus supplementary information to address whether it would be possible to set a target maximum for *trans* fat.

Reasons for Limiting Intakes of Fats and Cholesterol

Limiting the intakes of saturated fat, cholesterol, and *trans* fat helps support healthful blood lipids. Avoiding excessive total fat intake helps control saturated fat intake and helps avoid the intake of excessive calories. Adequate fat intake helps ensure adequate intake of vitamin E and essential fatty acids, helps support a normal pattern of growth, and may help avoid unfavorable changes in certain blood lipids (HHS/USDA, 2005).

Preliminary Targets for Total Fat, Saturated Fat, and Cholesterol

For children, *Dietary Guidelines for Americans* (HHS/USDA, 2005) recommends a fat intake of 25 to 35 percent of total calories, less than 10 percent of calories from saturated fatty acids (which are abundant in the fat in dairy products and meat), and a maximum of 300 mg of cholesterol per day for all individuals over the age of 2 years. The committee used these values as the basis for the preliminary fat targets for school meals.

trans Fat

Dietary Guidelines for Americans (HHS/USDA, 2005) recommends that *trans* fat intake be kept as low as possible, but it does not specify a maximum level of intake. In turn, no data exist on which to base a maximum level for *trans* fat in school meals, even though the goal is essentially zero grams. Nonetheless, a practical method can be used to keep the *trans* fat content of school meals to a minimum. In particular, this is achievable by specifying that, for any food included on the school menu (including any ingredient used by schools to prepare the food), 0 g of *trans* fat per serving would be the maximum amount of *trans* fat listed on the nutrition label or in manufacturer's specifications. This method is not always applicable because some products, such as bakery items produced by manufacturers who qualify as small businesses, are exempted from nutrition labeling, and thus the *trans* fat content of the product may not be specified. The committee notes that foods labeled as containing 0 g of *trans* fat may actually contain a small amount (< 0.5 g) of *trans* fat per serving. The rounding rules for declaring 0 g of *trans* fat are established based on analytical variance for the substance, and any amount that is rounded down to zero is considered "dietarily insignificant" by the Food and Drug Administration (FDA, 2008). Nonetheless, relying on label declarations is the only practical approach to keeping the *trans* fat content of school meals as close to zero as possible.

SETTING TARGETS FOR PROTEIN, VITAMINS, AND MINERALS

The report *Dietary Reference Intakes: Applications in Dietary Planning* (IOM, 2003) devotes a chapter to methods for planning daily diets for groups and discusses how to plan for a target usual nutrient intake distribution. In setting the preliminary nutrient targets for school meals, the committee followed these guidelines, adapting and modifying them as necessary to meet challenges described in Chapter 2. The work of this committee represents one of the first uses of the proposed dietary planning approach for a large national program and thus extends what was a theoretical approach to an important practical application. The challenges, and solutions, presented below should provide useful guidance to others wishing to set nutrient targets for similar purposes. They also indicate the need for further evaluation of the process, as indicated in the section "Recommendations for Evaluation" in Chapter 10.

Overview of the Target Median Intake Approach

The overall goal of planning intakes for groups of people, such as schoolchildren, is to achieve usual daily intakes within the group that meet the requirements of most individuals but are not excessive (IOM, 2003). This goal is accomplished by combining information on the group's usual nutrient intakes with information on the group's nutrient requirements (expressed as either Estimated Average Requirements or Adequate Intakes) and Tolerable Upper Intake Levels. The target nutrient intake distribution that is chosen aims to achieve the combined goal of a low predicted prevalence of nutrient inadequacy and a low predicted prevalence of excessive intakes. The median of this intake distribution is the *Target Median Intake*. The Target Median Intake is the starting point for the committee's calculations to derive the Nutrient Targets for school meals. The initial Target Median

Intakes for nutrients, which are discussed in the following two sections, appear in Appendix Table J-1.

Setting Targets for Nutrients with an Estimated Average Requirement

Overview

For most nutrients with an Estimated Average Requirement (EAR), the current prevalence of inadequacy may be estimated using the EAR cut-point method (IOM, 2006). If the prevalence of inadequacy is too high, then one goal of the planning process is to reduce the prevalence of inadequacy to an acceptable level. Thus, one of the steps in planning for the nutrient intake of groups is to select the target prevalence of inadequacy. The committee set 5 percent rather than the more conservative 2 to 3 percent that has been suggested as an acceptable level of inadequacy (IOM, 2003) for three reasons:

1. The intake distributions for school meal participants come from SNDA-III (USDA/FNS, 2007a). Although the overall sample of children was large, the number of children in specific age and gender groups was relatively small (approximately 200 to 300), and the standard errors in the tails of the distribution were large. Estimates at the 5th percentile were more stable than those at the 2.5th percentile and less likely to be affected by outliers.
2. Nutrient intakes collected using the 24-hour diet recall are likely to be underreported, especially by adolescent girls. Intakes in the bottom 2.5 percent of the distribution are very likely to be underestimates. As a result, using the 2.5th percentile as the basis for setting the Nutrition Standards might result in unnecessarily high standards.
3. Data were unavailable on the effect of changes in the school meals on the rest of the day's intake.

The EARs used to determine the Target Median Intakes for schoolchildren 6–10 years of age are weighted averages of two age groups. The use of weighted averages was necessary because the proposed elementary school group for school meals spans part of two Dietary Reference Intake (DRI) age groups (ages 4–8 and 9–13 years). The weighting factor was the proportion of the 5-year age span: three-fifths for ages 6–8 years and two-fifths for ages 9–10 years.

Description of the Method

To achieve a target nutrient intake distribution with approximately a 5 percent prevalence of inadequacy, it is necessary to alter the current distribution of children's intakes for many nutrients. Using the method recommended by the Institute of Medicine (IOM, 2003), the committee shifted each current intake distribution upward or downward until approximately 5 percent of the group's intakes were below the EAR. This method for determining the target distribution assumes that a change in the nutrient content of the daily diet would apply to everyone, and thus the distribution of usual nutrient intakes would shift without changing the shape of the distribution.[1] Under this assumption, the appropriate change in the nutrient intake distribution was calculated as follows:

- The 5th percentile of the intake distribution was positioned at the EAR.
- The new median of the distribution was calculated as the original median plus the difference between the intake at the 5th percentile and the EAR. If current intake at the 5th percentile of the current intake distribution is above the EAR, the new median would be below the current median. *The new median is the Target Median Intake for the day.*

The same method was used for all vitamins and minerals with an EAR, except for iron (see discussion of iron below). It was also used to determine a protein Target Median Intake in grams per kilogram of body weight (the units of the EAR for protein). To convert the value to grams of protein per day, it is necessary to assume a body weight for the children in each age-grade group. The committee used the SNDA-III body weights shown in Appendix Tables F-1 and F-2 for the midpoint ages in each age-grade group and averaged the weights for males and females. Although energy needs were based on body weights from the CDC growth charts because they are the reference standards for healthy children, the committee decided to base protein needs on the actual reported body weights from SNDA-III. Because the SNDA-III weights are higher than the CDC body weights, this method ensures that the protein targets cover almost all schoolchildren. The resulting average body weights were 29.3 kg for the kindergarten through grade 5 group, 51.1 kg for the grade 6 through 8 group, and 67.0 kg for the grade 9 through 12 group.

[1]The committee recognizes weaknesses of this assumption; however, the method provides useful estimates, and a superior alternative method has not been developed.

Example

To illustrate the method, the vitamin C Target Median Intake for high school students is used as an example.

1. The SNDA-III data show that vitamin C *intakes* at the 5th percentile are
   a. 32 mg per day for males and
   b. 19 mg per day for females ages 14–18 years (Appendix Table I-1).
2. The EARs for vitamin C are 63 and 56 mg per day, respectively. Thus,
   - the intake of the males needs to increase by 31 mg per day (63 mg minus 32 mg equals 31 mg),
   - the intake of the females needs to increase by 37 mg per day (56 mg minus 19 mg equals 37 mg).

As a result,

3. The Target Median Intake for the males would be 121 mg per day (90 mg [the current median intake] plus 31 mg equals 121 mg per day).
4. The Target Median Intake for the females would be 104 mg per day (67 mg [the current median intake] plus 37 mg equals 104 mg per day).

Iron as a Special Case

Because iron requirements are not normally distributed for menstruating females, the EAR cut-point method is not appropriate for calculating the Target Median Intakes for iron for females ages 11–13 and 14–18 years. Instead, the committee used a modeling approach based on the probability method (IOM, 2001b, pp. 205–208) for females in these two age groups (see Appendix I). The resulting Target Median Intakes were 15.5 mg per day for females ages 11–13 years and 15.9 mg per day for females ages 14–18 years.

Nutrients with an Adequate Intake

General Approach

Some nutrients have an Adequate Intake (AI) rather than an EAR. Based on guidance from the Institute of Medicine (IOM, 2003), the committee assumed that a low prevalence of inadequacy would result if the median of the usual intake distribution was at least equal to the AI. Thus, for five nutrients with an AI (calcium, potassium, fiber, linoleic acid, and α-linolenic acid), the Target Median Intake would be set at the AI. As was done with the EARs, weighted averages were used for the AIs for the youngest age group (6–10 years). Although the derivation of the AI differs substantially among these nutrients and among different age-gender groups, the AI is still the most appropriate type of DRI to use to set the Target Median Intake.

Exceptions

Sodium The approach used to address sodium did not involve setting a Target Median Intake. Instead, the committee agreed to set maximum daily targets for sodium that are based on the age-specific ULs for sodium. This decision was made for several reasons. The AI for sodium is 1.2 g per day for children ages 5–8 years and 1.5 g per day for older children—far less than children consume on average. Recognizing that sodium intake in the United States far exceeds the AI and also the Tolerable Upper Intake Level (UL), the sodium recommendation in *Dietary Guidelines for Americans* is 2.3 g per day—the value of the UL for persons ages 14 years and older. (The ULs for children younger than 14 years are slightly lower than 2.3 g per day.) Basing the sodium target on the UL rather than the AI is more consistent with achieving meals that are palatable and thus acceptable to U.S. schoolchildren. For sodium, the goal would be to reduce the median intake to the UL.

Vitamin D A Target Median Intake was not calculated for vitamin D (which has an AI) because of a lack of reliable data on the vitamin D content of foods and on vitamin D intakes. Vitamin D intakes were not assessed for SNDA-III. Although vitamin D intakes have recently been estimated for the What We Eat in America survey (NHANES 2005–2006) (USDA/ARS, 2009a) and were found to be low, especially for adolescent females, the age groups for the reported data could not be used to calculate Target Median Intakes for the age groups in this report.

Although exposure to sunshine reduces the need to ingest vitamin D, this vitamin D source is highly variable and is not under the control of school meal programs. Thus the role of sunshine in providing vitamin D was not considered by the committee. As described in the "Supportive Findings" section of Chapter 3, the committee is aware of the pending Institute of Medicine report on the requirements and upper levels of intake for vitamin D and acknowledges the appropriateness of using that report in the future to inform decisions that may be made about the vitamin D levels in school meals.

Method and Rationale for Calculating the School Meal-Target Median Intakes

To incorporate the Target Median Intake concept into the setting of the Nutrient Targets for school meals, the committee first addressed the fact that nutrient needs differ substantially between males and females within the age-grade groups. Its aim was to calculate targets for total daily intake that would best reflect these differences in nutrient needs. The committee used three methods of calculation (described below) to obtain candidate values for School Meal-Target Median Intakes (School Meal-TMIs). Regardless of the method used, the committee deemed the differences in requirements too small to consider both gender- and age-specific requirements within the grade group that encompasses kindergarten through grade 5. Thus, in examining the three approaches to setting School Meal-TMIs, only gender was considered within the kindergarten through grade 5 group.

Calculation Method Used

The committee used the following three methods to combine the Target Median Intakes by gender for each of the three grade groups.

1. *Average Target Median Intake.* Calculate the values for males and females separately within each of the grade groups (see Appendix Table J-1), and calculate the *average* for the grade group as the candidate School Meal-TMI.
2. *Highest Target Median Intake.* Calculate the values for males and females separately within each of the grade groups, and use the *higher one* for the grade group as the candidate School Meal-TMI.
3. *Simple Nutrient Density*[2] *Target Median Intake.* Calculate the nutrient density (the ratio of the gender-specific Target Median Intake to the gender-specific Estimated Energy Requirement shown in Table 2-4) for males and females separately within each of the grade groups. Then multiply the *higher density* times the mean Estimated Energy Requirement for the grade group to obtain the candidate School Meal-TMI.

The simple nutrient density method (#3 above) had been specifically designed for this purpose (IOM, 2003). Although other approaches have

[2]The term *nutrient density* has been used in different ways in the literature. The usage presented here is the one presented in *Dietary Reference Intakes: Applications in Dietary Planning* (IOM, 2003). This usage applies to setting a target for daily intake of each nutrient relative to daily calorie needs. In other sections of this report, the committee refers to the nutrient density of *foods* and has adopted the definition that it considers most useful and understandable: namely, the nutrient density of foods refers to the amount of a specific nutrient in a food per 100 calories of that food.

been proposed, they were considered unnecessarily complex for setting school meal targets. Nutrient density may be expressed in several ways; the approach described here considers each nutrient's requirement for a group of children relative to the energy requirement for the same group—that is, the ratio of the amount of a nutrient to the energy provided by the diet (IOM, 2003, p. 14).

Comparison of Results

The differences in the resulting candidate School Meal-TMI values from the three methods were not large, ranging up to 11 percent across 20 nutrients within the kindergarten through grade 5 group, up to 23 percent (for iron) within the grade 6 through 8 group, and up to 19 percent (for iron) within the grade 9 through 12 group (Appendix Table J-2). In general, the following conclusions can be drawn by comparing the results of the three methods.

- Calculating the average Target Median Intake usually resulted in the lowest value. This level of total *daily* intake, if achieved, should result in approximately a 5 percent *overall* prevalence of inadequacy for the grade group, but a higher than 5 percent prevalence for one of the gender groups. For example, females might have a higher than 5 percent prevalence of inadequacy, and males might have a prevalence of inadequacy of less than 5 percent.
- By comparison, the use of a School Meal-TMI based on the highest Target Median Intake would result in a *maximum* prevalence of inadequacy of 5 percent for either of the gender groups within the grade group. For example, females might have a 5 percent prevalence of inadequacy, but males would have a prevalence of less than 5 percent.
- The nutrient density method often results in the highest values, particularly for the two older grade groups. It sets the concentration of the nutrient high enough to result in a maximum of a 5 percent prevalence of inadequacy even if one of the gender groups has a lower energy requirement and thus consumes less food. Because energy requirements are similar for males and females in the kindergarten through grade 5 group, this method yields a value that is similar to the values obtained using the other methods for this age-grade group.

Example to Illustrate the Nutrient Density Method

Continuing with the vitamin C example above, the nutrient density of the requirements is calculated as the Target Median Intake divided by the

Estimated Energy Requirement (Table 2-4), as shown in equations *i* and *ii* below:

i. 120 mg vitamin C divided by 2,686 calories = 0.0448 mg/calorie for males and

ii. 104 mg divided by 2,044 calories = 0.0511 mg/calorie for females.

Because the nutrient density for vitamin C is higher for the females, the Target Median Intake based on nutrient density would be shown by equation *iii*:

iii. 0.0511 (the nutrient density) times 2,365 calories/day (the average Estimated Energy Requirement for males and females) = 121 mg per day.

As shown in equation *iii* above, the nutrient density is multiplied by the average Estimated Energy Requirement for males and females because the calories provided by the school meals reflect the average calorie needs of both genders. However, the nutrient density of the foods consumed should be high enough to cover the needs of the females in the likely event that their calorie intake is below this average. If the committee had assumed a sedentary level of activity rather than a light-active level for the older females, their lower Estimated Energy Requirements would have led to nutrient density Target Median Intakes that would be unrealistically high.[3] For youth ages 14–18 years, the vitamin C nutrient density Target Median Intake is similar to the values obtained using methods to calculate both the average and the highest Target Median Intake (see Appendix Table J-2), but that is not the case for a number of other nutrients (e.g., potassium).

Selection of the Nutrient Density Method

The committee chose the nutrient density method of setting the School Meal-TMIs. The committee notes that the nutrient density method aligns well with the emphasis placed on nutrient density by the *Dietary Guidelines*, where the focus is on selecting foods that provide substantial amounts of vitamins and minerals but relatively few calories. Using the simple nutrient

[3]Because calories enter the equations used for the nutrient density method, it may be helpful to recognize how the committee's early decision about calories would affect the results. In particular, what difference does it make when calorie needs for female adolescents are estimated using a low-active rather than a sedentary level of activity? In that case, the divisor in formula *i* would be smaller, meaning that the resulting nutrient density would be higher. Although it would be multiplied by a slightly lower average number of calories, the result would be a higher value for the School Meal-TMI.

density approach to set targets for each nutrient is likely to provide a basis for menus that correspond closely to the goals of the *Dietary Guidelines*.

Although the resulting School Meal-TMIs were often somewhat higher than those obtained from the other two methods, they represent the daily targets most likely to result in a low prevalence of inadequacy (5 percent or less) among the more vulnerable gender group (typically, the females). That is, the nutrient density method is designed to achieve a 5 percent prevalence of inadequacy for females even if the females' daily calorie intake is lower than the mean value set for the grade group.

Limitations of the Target Median Intake Methods

The Target Median Intake methodology makes several assumptions. An important one is that the additional amounts of nutrient in the diet will be consumed by everyone. That is, the shape of the intake distribution will not change. Although this assumption may not be correct, there is almost no evidence on which to base a different assumption. The research recommendations in Chapter 10 recognize this limitation and call for more research on this topic. Likewise, although the Target Median Intake approach is designed for setting daily nutrient targets, the school meals can only alter intakes at specific meals. The impact on the rest of the day's intake is unknown. Moreover, the students themselves determine how much of the school meal they will consume. Thus, it is not possible to conclude that Nutrient Targets based on the selected School Meal-TMI will result in a low prevalence of nutrient inadequacy for the total day's intake. However, the nutrient density School Meal-TMI is based on the methodology recommended in the DRI planning report (IOM, 2003), and the resulting nutrient targets represent a step forward in applying the DRIs to planning intakes for groups so as to reduce the prevalence of inadequate nutrient intakes.

DAILY SCHOOL MEAL-TARGET MEDIAN INTAKES COMPARED WITH MYPYRAMID FOOD PATTERNS

The final School Meal-TMIs are the values obtained using the nutrient density approach. For these values to be useful, they need to correspond well with daily food patterns that meet *Dietary Guidelines*. To address this, the committee compared the daily School Meal-TMIs with the nutrient content of the corresponding MyPyramid food patterns (Table 4-4). For almost all nutrients, the School Meal-TMI value was lower than the amount of the nutrient that would be obtained by following the MyPyramid pattern. This means that MyPyramid food patterns provide a sound basis for developing standards for menu planning. For the youngest age group (ages 5–10 years), vitamin E and potassium are the only nutrients that would be provided

TABLE 4-4 Daily SM-TMIs[a] for Different Age Groups Compared to MyPyramid Food Intake Patterns

	6–10 y, 1,800-Calorie Intake Pattern			11–13 y, 2,000-Calorie Intake Pattern			14–18 y, 2,400-Calorie Intake Pattern		
Nutrient	SM-TMI	1,800 calories/d MyPyramid Pattern*	MyPyramid Nutrient as % of SM-TMI	SM-TMI	2,000 calories/d MyPyramid Pattern*	MyPyramid Nutrient as % of SM-TMI	SM-TMI	2,400 calories/d MyPyramid Pattern*	MyPyramid Nutrient as % of SM-TMI
Protein (g/d)[b]	47.4	87	184	100.6	91	90	101.6	105	103
Vitamin A (μg RAE/d)	601	1011	168	753	1,052	140	867	1126	130
Vitamin C (mg/d)	74	130	176	93	155	167	121	163	135
Vitamin E (mg αT/d)	9.3	8.6	92	12.5	9.5	76	17	10.7	63
Thiamin (mg/d)	1.16	1.9	164	1.48	2.0	135	1.74	2.4	138
Riboflavin (mg/d)	1.45	2.7	186	1.9	2.8	147	2.08	3.1	149
Niacin (mg/d)	14.7	20.8	141	18.8	22	116	22.7	27.3	120
Vitamin B_6 (mg/d)	1.24	2.3	185	1.69	2.4	142	1.97	2.9	147
Folate (μg DFE/d)	425	668	157	528	695	132	640	822	128
Vitamin B_{12} (μg /d)	3.7	8.0	216	4.2	8.3	198	5.1	9.2	180
Iron (mg/d)	10.5	17	162	16.4[c]	17.5	107	18.4[c]	21.5	117
Magnesium (mg/d)	226	363	161	306	390	127	459	440	96
Zinc (mg/d)	9.1	13.7	151	11.6	14.3	123	13.5	16.7	124
Calcium (mg/d)	1,037	1,302	126	1,375	1,316	96	1,504	1,388	92
Phosphorus (mg/d)	1,127	1,691	150	1,682	1,740	103	1,787	1,961	110
Potassium (mg/d)	4,229	3,784	89	4,760	4,044	85	5,438	4,416	81
Linoleic Acid (g)	10.4	15.9	153	11.4	18	155	14.1	20.9	148
α-Linolenic Acid (g)	0.97	1.6	165	1.14	2	149	1.41	2	143
Fiber (g/d)	26.5	29	109	29.4	31	105	33.5	37	110

NOTES: αT = α-tocopherol; d = day; DFE = dietary folate equivalent; g = gram; kg = kilogram; mg = milligram; RAE = retinol activity equivalents; SM-TMI = School Meal-Target Median Intake; μg = micrograms; y = years.

[a]Sodium is excluded from this table because the SM-TMI approach was not used to set the target for this nutrient.

[b]Assumes body weights of 29.3 kg for children ages 6–10 years, 51.1 kg for children ages 11–13 years, and 67.0 kg for children ages 14–18 years (average body weights from Tables F-1 and F-2 in Appendix F).

[c]Iron values were based on results of calculations that used the probability method. Details appear in Appendix I.

SOURCE: *Britten et al., 2006. Reprinted from *Journal of Nutrition Education and Behavior*, 38/6 Supp., P. Britten, K. Marcoe, S. Yamini, and C. Davis, Development of Food Intake Patterns for the MyPyramid Food Guidance System, pp. S78–S92, Copyright (2006), with permission from Elsevier.

by the MyPyramid pattern in amounts below the School Meal-TMI. For the middle school group (ages 11–13 years), these same two nutrients, as well as calcium and protein intakes, would be somewhat below the School Meal-TMI. For the high school group (ages 14–18 years), the amount of vitamin E provided by the MyPyramid pattern would be only 63 percent of the School Meal-TMI; potassium would be about 80 percent of the target; calcium and magnesium would be slightly below the targets.

CONVERTING DAILY SCHOOL MEAL-TARGET MEDIAN INTAKES TO BREAKFAST AND LUNCH NUTRIENT TARGETS

School Meal-TMIs are for daily intake, but school meals provide only a portion of the day's intake. As described earlier in this chapter, the committee set a preliminary range of calories for school breakfast (19 to 24 percent of the day's total) and for school lunch (30 to 34 percent of the day's total). When developing recommendations for the Nutrient Targets for school meals, the committee multiplied the School Meal-TMIs, the maximum for cholesterol, and the sodium ULs by the midpoint of those percentages to obtain *preliminary* nutrient targets. That is, the targets for breakfast represent 21.5 percent of the School Meal-TMIs, and the targets for lunch represent 32 percent. Preliminary nutrient targets for school meals appear in Table 4-5.

The committee recognizes that school food authorities have no way to ensure that students will achieve the target nutrient intake distribution for the day or even the Nutrient Targets for school meals. The target nutrient intake distribution would be achieved only if students' intake from school meals were accompanied by similar changes in the nutrient intakes from foods consumed *outside* the school meal setting. That is, the recommended amounts of nutrients from the school meals would need to be consumed, and comparable intakes would have to be sustained across the full day's intake in order to meet the School Meal-TMI and achieve a 5 percent prevalence of inadequacy. Nonetheless, it is desirable to set Nutrient Targets for school meals to provide a scientific basis for standards for menu planning and also to serve as a model for the meals and snacks served outside the school meal setting.

CONSIDERATION OF THE TOLERABLE UPPER INTAKE LEVEL IN THE SETTING OF NUTRIENT TARGETS

The committee examined the possibility that, for some nutrients, the prevalence of intakes above the UL would be undesirably high if the School Meal-TMIs were achieved for the full day's intake. Data from SNDA-III for children ages 6–18 years were used for this purpose. An "adjusted" intake

TABLE 4-5 Preliminary Nutrient Targets for Selected Nutrients, by Meal and Age Group

	Breakfast[a]			Lunch[b]		
Nutrient (unit)	5–10 y	11–13 y	14–18 y	5–10 y	11–13 y	14–18 y
Calories (kcal)	350–450	400–500	450–600	550–650	600–700	700–800
Cholesterol (mg)*	< 65	< 65	< 65	< 96	< 96	< 96
Total fat (% of kcal)*	25–35	25–35	25–35	25–35	25–35	25–35
Saturated fat (% of kcal)*	< 10	< 10	< 10	< 10	< 10	< 10
trans fat (g/d)	NA[c]	NA[c]	NA[c]	NA[c]	NA[c]	NA[c]
Linoleic acid (g/d)	2.2	2.5	3.0	3.3	3.6	4.5
α-Linolenic acid (g/d)	0.21	0.25	0.30	0.31	0.36	0.45
Protein (g/d)	10.2	21.6	21.8	15.2	32.2	32.5
Vitamin A (μg RAE/d)	129	162	186	192	241	277
Vitamin C (mg/d)	16	20	26	24	30	39
Vitamin E (mg αT/d)	2.0	2.7	3.7	3.0	4.0	5.4
Thiamin (mg/d)	0.2	0.3	0.4	0.4	0.5	0.6
Riboflavin (mg/d)	0.31	0.41	0.45	0.46	0.61	0.67
Niacin (mg/d)	3.2	4.0	4.9	4.7	6.0	7.3
Vitamin B_6 (mg/d)	0.3	0.4	0.4	0.4	0.5	0.6
Folate (μg DFE/d)	91	114	138	136	169	205
Vitamin B_{12} (μg/d)	0.8	0.9	1.1	1.2	1.3	1.6
Iron (mg/d)	2.3	3.5	4.0	3.4	5.2	5.9
Magnesium (mg/d)	49	66	99	72	98	147
Zinc (mg/d)	2.0	2.5	2.9	2.9	3.7	4.3
Calcium (mg/d)	223	296	323	332	440	481
Phosphorus (mg/d)	242	362	384	361	538	572
Potassium (mg/d)	909	1,023	1,169	1,353	1,523	1,740
Sodium (mg/d)[d]	≤ 434	≤ 473	≤ 495	≤ 636	≤ 704	≤ 736
Fiber (g/d)	5.7	6.3	7.2	8.5	9.4	10.7

NOTES: αT = α-tocopherol; d = day; DFE = dietary folate equivalent; g = gram; kg = kilogram; mg = milligram; RAE = retinol activity equivalent; μg = microgram; y = years.

[a]Targets based on 21.5 percent of the daily School Meal-Target Median Intake for the age-grade group.

[b]Targets based on 32 percent of the daily School Meal-Target Median Intake for the age-grade group.

[c]Zero grams of *trans* fat per serving as listed on the nutrition label or in manufacturer's specifications, for any food included on the school menu.

[d]Targets for sodium, which are based on the Tolerable Upper Intake Level, are for the year 2020.

SOURCE: *HHS/USDA, 2005.

at the 95th percentile was calculated assuming that the median intake of a nutrient changed to be equal to the School Meal-TMI and that the whole distribution (including the 95th percentile) would change by the same amount. Calculations were performed separately for males and females within each grade group. This same method was used for nutrients with an EAR and for nutrients with an AI.

For each of the three age-grade groups covered by the SNDA-III data (6–10, 11–13, and 14–18 years), the adjusted intake at the 95th percentile was compared to the UL. (Magnesium was excluded because the UL is only for pharmacological agents. The UL does not apply to magnesium in foods [IOM, 1997].) For children ages 6–10 years, the UL for the younger children (ages 6–8 years)—that is, the most conservative value—was used. For several nutrients, the ULs are considerably lower for children ages 8 years or younger than for the older children.

The results are shown in Table 4-6. For each grade group, there were some nutrients with the adjusted 95th percentile of intakes above the UL, meaning that at least 5 percent of the children would have intakes above the UL if the median intake was at the School Meal-TMI, as follows

- 6–10-year-olds: vitamin A, niacin, folate, and zinc for males and females
- 11–13-year-olds: niacin and folate for males and females
- 14–18-year-olds: niacin and folate for males and females; males' 95th percentile of intake would be slightly above the calcium UL

It is worth noting that in all these cases except calcium, current intakes at the 95th percentile also exceed the UL. As would be expected, at the 95th percentile of intake, all values for sodium are well above the UL.

For most nutrients, intakes above the UL are not likely to be a concern. This is largely because the ULs only apply to certain forms or sources of nutrients, whereas the intake estimates are for the total diet. The degree of concern about intakes above the UL is summarized for six nutrients below.

- **Probably a concern**

  Sodium 50 percent of schoolchildren would have intakes above the sodium UL. See Chapter 3 regarding effects of sodium on blood pressure. Nonetheless, setting the School Meal-TMI to *reduce* intakes to less than the UL is a reasonable goal.
- **Probably not a concern**

  Vitamin A The UL applies only to preformed vitamin A (retinol). Dairy products and eggs are the most common sources of preformed vitamin A in children's diets. It would take approximately 1.5 quarts of milk to exceed the UL for children ages 5–8 years, and much more than that for the older children.

  Calcium Although the adjusted intakes for the older males might result in 5 percent with intakes above the calcium UL, the committee agreed

TABLE 4-6 Tolerable Upper Intake Level (UL) for Nutrients with a UL,* Reported Intakes,**,[a] Predicted Adjusted Intakes at the 95th Percentile, and Adjusted Intakes as a Percentage of the UL, by Age-Gender Group

Nutrient (unit)	UL[b]	Intake at 95th	Adj. Intake at 95th	Adj. Intake as % of UL	UL[b]	Intake at 95th	Adj. Intake at 95th	Adj. Intake as % of UL
	Males				Females			
	6–10 years				6–10 years			
Vitamin A (μg RAE/d)	900	**1,025**	**1,010**	112	900	**1,022**	**1,024**	114
Vitamin C (mg/d)	650	169	162	25	650	161	146	22
Vitamin E (mg αT/d)	300	7.5	11.1	4	300	8.9	13.3	4
Niacin (mg/d)	15.0	**29.3**	**23.9**	159	15.0	**30.9**	**26.1**	174
Vitamin B_6 (mg/d)	40	2.4	2.0	5	40	2.6	2.3	6
Folate (μg DFE/d)	400	**951**	**834**	209	400	**988**	**887**	222
Iron (mg/d)	40	24	20	50	40	24	21	52
Zinc (mg/d)	12	**17.4**	**15.5**	129	12	**16.7**	**15.9**	133
Calcium (mg/d)	2,500	1,927	1,863	75	2,500	1,579	1,571	63
Phosphorus (mg/d)	3,000	2,027	1,753	58	3,000	1,708	1,531	51
Sodium (mg/d)	1,900	**4,661**	**3,321**	175	1,900	**4,405**	**3,249**	171
	11–13 years				11–13 years			
Vitamin A (μg RAE/d)	1,700	1,225	1,314	77	1,700	1,006	1,254	74
Vitamin C (mg/d)	1,200	181	185	15	1,200	164	187	16
Vitamin E (mg αT/d)	600	10.4	16.8	3	600	11.5	19	3
Niacin (mg/d)	20.0	**35.0**	**31.9**	160	20.0	**31.6**	**31.4**	157
Vitamin B_6 (mg/d)	60	3.5	3.4	6	60	2.7	2.9	5
Folate (μg DFE/d)	600	**1,081**	**986**	164	600	**994**	**1,062**	177
Iron (mg/d)	40	25	25.2	63	40	25	27.7	69
Zinc (mg/d)	23	18.2	17.8	77	23	16.3	18.4	80
Calcium (mg/d)	2,500	1,724	1,926	77	2,500	1,612	2,128	85
Phosphorus (mg/d)	4,000	1,984	2,236	56	4,000	1,925	2,489	62
Sodium (mg/d)	2,200	**5,180**	**3,599**	164	2,200	**5,028**	**3,970**	180

	14–18 years				14–18 years			
Vitamin A (µg RAE/d)	2,800	1,238	1,509	54	2,800	914	1,380	49
Vitamin C (mg/d)	1,800	207	244	14	1,800	186	246	14
Vitamin E (mg αT/d)	800	12	22.6	3	800	10.6	23.1	3
Niacin (mg/d)	30.0	**40.1**	**36.7**	122	30.0	**30.2**	**35.7**	119
Vitamin B_6 (mg/d)	80	3.2	3.1	4	80	2.6	3.3	4
Folate (µg DFE/d)	800	**1,216**	**1,238**	155	800	**948**	**1,175**	147
Iron (mg/d)	45	31.3	31.8	71	45	23.6	30.2	67
Zinc (mg/d)	34	24.1	24	7	34	16	21	62
Calcium (mg/d)	2,500	2,134	**2,519**	101	2,500	1,482	2,251	90
Phosphorus (mg/d)	4,000	2,530	2,775	69	4,000	1,809	2,589	65
Sodium (mg/d)	2,300	**6,280**	**4,072**	177	2,300	**4,558**	**3,690**	160

NOTES: αT = α-tocopherol; Adj. = Adjusted; d = day; DFE = dietary folate equivalent; g = gram; kg = kilogram; mg = milligram; RAE = retinol activity equivalent; µg = microgram. Bold font indicates intake values above the UL.

[a]Intakes exclude contributions from nutrient supplements. Magnesium is excluded from the table because the UL for magnesium applies only to pharmacological agents.

[b]The UL listed is the lowest UL value within the age-grade group.

SOURCES: *IOM, 2006; **USDA/FNS, 2007a.

that these very high calcium intakes were not likely to be a result of intakes from school meals and thus would not be a concern when setting the School Meal-TMI for calcium for the oldest grade group.

Zinc. The UL for children ages 4–8 years is very low, and it may be more applicable to children ages 4–5 years than to children ages 6–8 years (Zlotkin, 2006).

- **Unknown concern**

Niacin The UL applies only to niacin from supplements and from foods that are fortified with niacin. The committee notes that it is not known if highly fortified foods (such as those that provide 100 percent of the Daily Value for niacin [20 mg] in a single serving) pose a risk for young children. Although this amount exceeds the UL for niacin for the youngest children and equals the UL for children ages 11–13 years, many children's intakes are already at this level. The ULs for children were based on limited evidence that some adults experienced flushing as a short-term response to the ingestion of high levels of nicotinic acid (a form of niacin that does not occur naturally in foods and that differs from niacinamide, which is the substance used to fortify foods) (IOM, 1998).

Folate Current intakes at the 95th percentile exceed the folate UL for all grade and gender groups. The adjusted intake distributions would result in intakes that exceed the UL for three of the age-gender groups, especially the youngest grade groups; but intakes for the other three age-gender groups would probably be below the UL (Table 4-6). The UL applies only to synthetic forms of folic acid (e.g., the folic acid added to fortify enriched grains, not the folate that occurs naturally in foods). The 95th percentile intakes, however, would be almost twice the UL for the youngest children. It is not known if highly fortified foods (such as those that provide 100 percent of the Daily Value for folate [400 μg] in a single serving; an amount that equals the UL for the younger children) pose a risk for young children. As is the case with niacin, the ULs for folate for children were based on limited evidence from studies with adults; but, in this case, they were *long-term* studies on folic acid ingestion (IOM, 1998).

CHAPTER SUMMARY

The Nutrient Targets are intended to serve as a guide for setting standards for menu planning, not for direct use in menu planning. This made it reasonable for the committee to develop targets for 24 nutrients. The committee used a data-based method to set preliminary minimum and maximum target calorie levels for school breakfast and lunch for the three age-grade groups, rounding the values for ease of implementation. Setting both a minimum and a maximum level has the advantages of providing adequate intake without encouraging the overconsumption of calories, while still allowing some flexibility to school food service operators. The committee based its preliminary targets for saturated fat, cholesterol, and total fat on *Dietary Guidelines for Americans* and used a labeling approach to address *trans* fat.

In setting the preliminary nutrient targets for protein, vitamins, and minerals, the committee used methods recommended by the Institute of Medicine for using the DRIs in planning for groups. The use of the nutrient density method results in nutrient targets that recognize that females have nutrient needs that ordinarily are higher than those of males relative to their calorie needs. Thus, the resulting Nutrient Targets should provide a sound basis for planning menus that are appropriate for both males and females in the age-grade group. Although the resulting intakes at the 95th percentile may exceed the UL for some nutrients, especially for the youngest children, it is unlikely that the amounts provided by the school meals pose a health risk.

5

Process for Developing the Meal Requirements

Meal Requirements encompasses standards for school meals that are used for two purposes: (1) to develop menus that are consistent with *Dietary Guidelines* and the Nutrient Targets and (2) to specify what qualifies as a meal that is eligible for federal financial reimbursement. Meal Requirements comprise standards for meals *as offered* by the school and standards for meals *as selected*[1] by students. *As offered* meal standards are applied in the development of menus for school breakfast and lunch and thus may be called *standards for menu planning*. *As selected* meal standards are used by the cashier to determine whether the student has selected a meal that meets requirements for reimbursement. The process used by the committee to develop the Meal Requirements was iterative in nature, and it also contributed to the committee's final recommendations for the Nutrient Targets. This chapter describes the processes used to develop recommendations for the Meal Requirements. Different processes were used to develop the standards for menu planning and for meals *as selected*. The final recommendations appear in Chapter 7.

DEVELOPMENT OF STANDARDS FOR MENU PLANNING

The development of standards for menu planning involved five major steps: (1) consideration of the adequacy of the meal planning approaches in current use; (2) the selection of the new meal planning approach; (3) the identification of an established food pattern guide to serve as a basis for

[1]Currently called standards for meals *as served*.

school meal patterns for planning menus that are consistent with *Dietary Guidelines for Americans*; (4) the design and use of spreadsheets to test possible meal patterns against the preliminary nutrition targets established in Chapter 4; and (5) the testing of a series of possible standards for menu planning and evaluation of the resulting menus in terms of nutrient content, cost, and suitability for school meals. These steps are described briefly below. Appendix H describes the third and fourth steps in more detail.

Consideration of Current Menu Planning Approaches

The two major categories of menu planning in current use are food-based menu planning and nutrient-based menu planning.

1. A food-based approach relies on the use of an approved meal pattern to serve as the basis for menu planning. The pattern specifies that the menu must include minimum amounts of food from selected food groups. The approach does not require the use of computer analysis to ensure that the existing Nutrient Standards are met, but some school food authorities (SFAs) supplement their food-based approach by conducting computerized analysis of some nutrients. Food-based approaches are the most common method of menu planning in current use (USDA/FNS, 2007a).
2. A nutrient-based approach focuses on nutrients rather than food groups. The menu planner uses a computerized process to ensure that the nutrient content of the menus conforms to the existing Nutrition Standards. The method does not include any food group specifications other than fluid milk. Two evaluations of nutrient-based menu planning (USDA/FNS, 1997, 1998a) revealed challenges related to staff resources, time requirements, and the software used but reported that the approach offered increased flexibility in menu planning. The resulting menus tended to be lower in saturated fat than they had been before the approach was adopted and tended to meet the existing Nutrition Standards for protein, two vitamins, and two minerals. Student participation rates and program costs remained about the same.

Development of a New Meal Planning Approach

A major component of the committee's task was to make recommendations for menu planning that would improve the consistency of school meals with both the *Dietary Guidelines* and the Dietary Reference Intakes (DRIs). Although the nutrient-based approach has certain advantages, the committee identified two serious limitations of this menu planning approach:

1. Analysis of an expanded list of nutrients (the preliminary nutrient targets [see Table 4-5] rather than the current five nutrients) would be needed because there is little evidence of "key" nutrients that would ensure an overall nutritionally adequate diet. This larger set of nutrients would create practical problems for the nutrient-based approach because of limited food composition data for many foods used in school meals and because the necessary software is not available to the school food authorities.

2. A focus on nutrients alone does not ensure alignment with the *Dietary Guidelines* recommendations, which place a strong emphasis on foods; and it may, in some cases, lead to unnecessary reliance on specially fortified foods.

Using solely a food-based meal planning approach, the foods offered could be made more consistent with *Dietary Guidelines* recommendations, and the meal pattern could be designed to be reasonably consistent with the DRIs for protein, nine vitamins, six minerals, fiber, and linoleic and α-linolenic acids (as illustrated in Chapter 3). However, a food-based approach alone would not be sufficient because it would not ensure that menus are appropriate in calorie content and meet *Dietary Guidelines* recommendations for saturated fat and sodium. Therefore, the committee concluded that a combined meal planning approach—one that is food based but that also incorporates specifications for a small number of dietary components—was needed to improve consistency with both the *Dietary Guidelines* and the DRIs. Although the committee considered more complex approaches that required additional nutrient analyses, it determined that a well-specified menu pattern precluded the need for such analyses.

Identification of a Food Pattern to Guide School Meal Planning

In response to comments on the Phase I report (IOM, 2008), the committee considered two food pattern guides to serve as a basis for the school meal patterns: the Thrifty Food Plan (USDA/CNPP, 2007) and the MyPyramid food intake patterns (USDA, 2005). The Thrifty Food Plan was designed for planning a minimal cost, healthful diet. The first constraint in developing the plan was cost (USDA/CNPP, 2007). The plan incorporates consumption patterns of low-income families and is consistent with *Dietary Guidelines*. The committee decided against its use for two reasons. In particular, (1) the Thrifty Food Plan makes use of 7 major food groups but a total of 58 food categories—an unwieldy number for SFAs to use for menu planning purposes; and (2) several categories of food listed under the plan's "other" group (ready-to-serve and condensed soups, dry soups, and frozen or refrigerated entrées [including pizza, fish sticks, and frozen meals]) are foods that are used frequently in many school meal programs. (The nutrient profiles of the "other" foods used by school meal programs tend to be more favorable than those of similar foods included in the Thrifty Food Plan.)

As described in Chapter 3 and in more detail in the Phase I report (IOM, 2008), the MyPyramid food intake patterns provide a basis for planning menus for a day that are consistent with the *Dietary Guidelines* and that provide nutrients in amounts that equal or exceed the most current Recommended Dietary Allowances—with two exceptions (vitamin E and potassium). The MyPyramid patterns specify amounts of foods from six major food groups and seven food subgroups—a larger number of food groups than currently used for planning school meals[2] but a number judged workable by the committee. To ensure that the nutrient amounts provided by the MyPyramid patterns would meet the School Meal-Target Median Intakes (School Meal-TMIs), the committee compared School Meal-TMIs for the elementary school, middle school, and high school age-grade groups with the nutrient content of MyPyramid patterns for 1,800, 2,000, and 2,400 calories (see Table 4-6 in Chapter 4). The School Meal-TMI values are less than 100 percent of the amounts of the nutrients in the MyPyramid patterns except for vitamin E and potassium for all age-grade levels, protein and calcium for schoolchildren ages 11 years and older, and also magnesium for schoolchildren ages 14 years and older.

MenuDevelopment Spreadsheets

The committee developed spreadsheets (called MenuDevelopment spreadsheets) to assist in designing and evaluating preliminary meal patterns for school breakfast and lunch. Upon entering test values for a meal pattern (the number of servings[3] from each food category per week), formulas in the spreadsheets calculate an estimate of the average daily nutrient content of the pattern and show how the nutrient estimates compare with the preliminary targets (preliminary nutrient targets are given in Table 4-7 in Chapter 4). These spreadsheets primarily used the 2005 MyPyramid nutrient composites (Marcoe et al., 2006) to estimate the energy and nutrient content that would be provided by possible meal patterns for breakfast and lunch. Modifications to the nutrient composites to make them more suitable for school meals are indicated in footnotes to Table H-2 in Appendix H. Figure 5-1 shows a portion of the spreadsheet for school lunch for ages 5–10 years (kindergarten through grade 5). The committee recognizes that the estimates obtained using the MenuDevelopment spreadsheets are

[2]Existing rules for food-based menu planning specify four food groups: (1) fluid milk, (2) meat/meat alternate, (3) vegetable/fruit, and (4) grain/bread.

[3]Careful attention was given to the amounts that are specified in MyPyramid, which refers to amounts rather than servings.

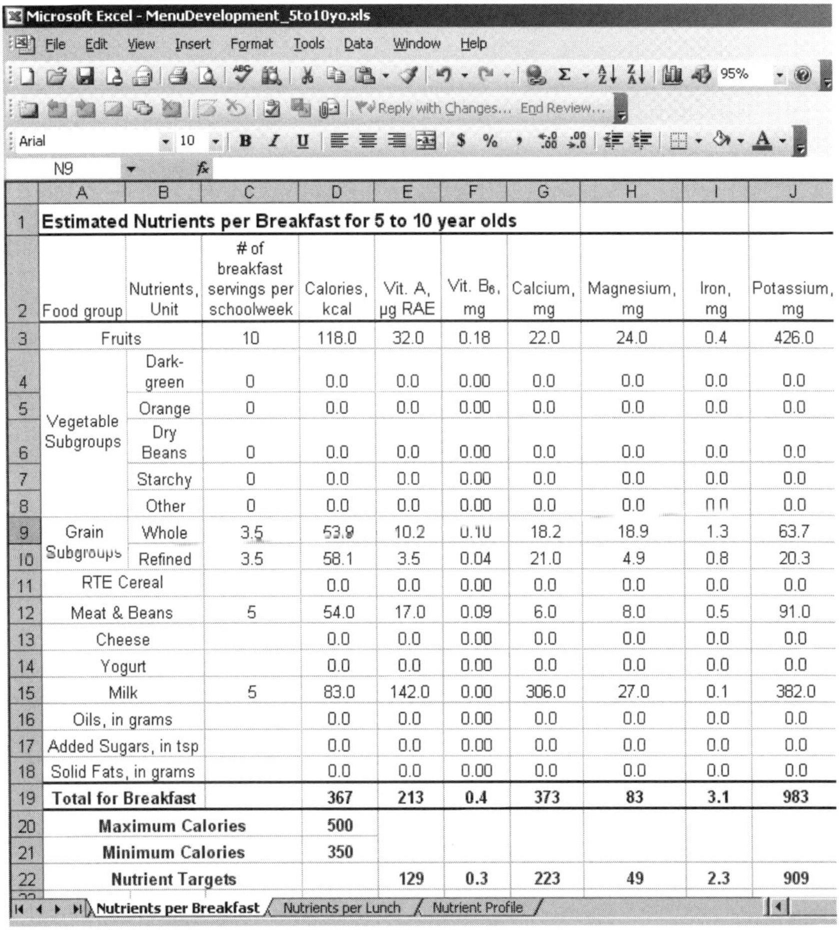

Microsoft Excel - MenuDevelopment_5to10yo.xls

	A	B	C	D	E	F	G	H	I	J
1	**Estimated Nutrients per Breakfast for 5 to 10 year olds**									
2	Food group	Nutrients, Unit	# of breakfast servings per schoolweek	Calories, kcal	Vit. A, µg RAE	Vit. B_6, mg	Calcium, mg	Magnesium, mg	Iron, mg	Potassium, mg
3	Fruits		10	118.0	32.0	0.18	22.0	24.0	0.4	426.0
4	Vegetable Subgroups	Dark-green	0	0.0	0.0	0.00	0.0	0.0	0.0	0.0
5		Orange	0	0.0	0.0	0.00	0.0	0.0	0.0	0.0
6		Dry Beans	0	0.0	0.0	0.00	0.0	0.0	0.0	0.0
7		Starchy	0	0.0	0.0	0.00	0.0	0.0	0.0	0.0
8		Other	0	0.0	0.0	0.00	0.0	0.0	0.0	0.0
9	Grain Subgroups	Whole	3.5	53.9	10.2	0.10	18.2	18.9	1.3	63.7
10		Refined	3.5	58.1	3.5	0.04	21.0	4.9	0.8	20.3
11	RTE Cereal			0.0	0.0	0.00	0.0	0.0	0.0	0.0
12	Meat & Beans		5	54.0	17.0	0.09	6.0	8.0	0.5	91.0
13	Cheese			0.0	0.0	0.00	0.0	0.0	0.0	0.0
14	Yogurt			0.0	0.0	0.00	0.0	0.0	0.0	0.0
15	Milk		5	83.0	142.0	0.00	306.0	27.0	0.1	382.0
16	Oils, in grams			0.0	0.0	0.00	0.0	0.0	0.0	0.0
17	Added Sugars, in tsp			0.0	0.0	0.00	0.0	0.0	0.0	0.0
18	Solid Fats, in grams			0.0	0.0	0.00	0.0	0.0	0.0	0.0
19	**Total for Breakfast**			**367**	**213**	**0.4**	**373**	**83**	**3.1**	**983**
20	**Maximum Calories**			**500**						
21	**Minimum Calories**			**350**						
22	**Nutrient Targets**				**129**	**0.3**	**223**	**49**	**2.3**	**909**

Nutrients per Breakfast / Nutrients per Lunch / Nutrient Profile

FIGURE 5-1 Excerpt from a late version of the MenuDevelopment spreadsheet for estimating and evaluating the average daily energy and nutrient content that would be provided by possible meal patterns for breakfast, using preliminary targets for schoolchildren ages 5–10 years (kindergarten through grade 5). The spreadsheet had been revised during the iteration period to include separate rows for low-fat cheese and low-fat sweetened yogurt (see Chapter 6). Added sugars and solid fats are included for testing purposes; they were not intended to be part of the menu pattern.

NOTES: The MenuDevelopment spreadsheet provides nutrient output for an additional 21 nutrients. Information about the food groups and nutrient composites used can be found in Appendix Table H-2. The "servings" refer to the amounts of food as specified in Appendix Table H-1. The use of unsaturated oils is encouraged within calorie limits.

approximations. The nutrient composites were designed using food consumption data from adults as well as children. Nonetheless, the committee considers them to be good approximations that help to design and test for nutritionally sound meal patterns.

School Meal Pattern Development

To begin developing the meal patterns, the committee assigned amounts of food from each MyPyramid food group to breakfast and lunch using the percentage of calories assigned for each meal. That is, for each age-grade group, the initial breakfast and lunch patterns (Table H-3 in Appendix H) were designed to correspond to approximately 21.5 percent of the MyPyramid amounts for breakfast and 32 percent of the MyPyramid amounts for lunch. This method keeps the food group amounts proportional to the number of calories specified for the meal. Because it is uncommon for a majority of U.S. schoolchildren to consume vegetables at breakfast (with a few exceptions, such as hash-brown potatoes), the committee agreed to omit all vegetables from the trial breakfast patterns and to test the effects of adding more fruit at breakfast.

The patterns were adjusted up or down if necessary to achieve practical serving amounts. For example, instead of specifying 0.8 cups of vegetable per day, ¾ cup or 1 cup would be specified. As work progressed, meal patterns were adjusted to consider student acceptance and school meal operations. (These topics are addressed further in Chapter 6.)

Because the foods specified by MyPyramid are the lowest fat forms and are free of added sugars, it was necessary to take discretionary calories (calories primarily from saturated fat and added sugars) into account during the testing with the MenuDevelopment spreadsheets. An allocation as made for the added sugars in flavored fat-free milk, for example, because retaining this type of milk in school meals is one way to promote milk intake by students (Garey et al., 1990). Although tentative allocations were made for discretionary calories from added sugars and saturated fat components, they were not intended to be part of any meal pattern.

Setting Additional Specifications

In working with the MenuDevelopment spreadsheets, it became obvious that three specifications from the preliminary nutrient targets would need to be an integral part of the standards for menu planning (that is, for meals *as offered*): (1) the minimum and maximum calorie level, (2) the limit on saturated fat, and (3) the maximum level of sodium. Simply specifying the number of servings to include from each of the food groups would not ensure that the meals would meet those targets. Evidence from the third

School Nutrition Dietary Assessment study (SNDA-III) makes it clear that calories, saturated fat, and sodium merit special attention. Thus the committee considered these additional dietary components when developing the standards for menu planning. The levels of total fat were consistently below 35 percent of calories when calories and saturated fat were controlled.

The committee notes that its approach to developing the standards for menu planning leaves relatively few discretionary calories for added sugars and saturated fat. In conjunction with the meal patterns, the specification of a maximum calorie level places limits on the use of foods with added sugars. This is quite consistent with the new recommendation from the American Heart Association (AHA) (Johnson et al., 2009) to limit added sugars to about half of the discretionary calorie allowance. With careful menu planning, enough discretionary calories should be available to cover flavored fat-free milk in place of plain fat-free milk as a daily option, some flavored low-fat yogurt, and some sweetened ready-to-eat cereals. These are highly nutritious foods that are very popular with many schoolchildren and that are identified in the AHA statement as potentially having a positive impact on diet quality. Fruits in light syrup contain about 10 grams of added sugars per half cup serving.[4] The omission of those sweetened foods might result in decreased student participation as well as in reduced nutrient intakes.

Testing of Revisions of Standards for Menu Planning

To test revisions of the standards for menu planning, the committee used two methods:

1. revision of representative baseline menus to determine the types of changes needed to meet new standards, followed by analysis of modified baseline menus to allow comparison of the nutrients, key food groups, and cost before and after the revision; and
2. writing sample menus to meet the revised standards.

This section describes both of these methods. The iterative nature of the methods is addressed in Chapter 6.

Analysis was conducted using a software application called the School Meals Menu Analysis (SMMA) program (see Appendix K), which was designed for this project at Iowa State University. After the data were entered in the program, the application allowed the estimation of the average daily (1) content of energy and 23 nutrients and (2) food cost for each set of

[4]Although fresh fruit would be preferable, canned fruit might be used for reasons such as cost, availability, and labor.

5-day menus. The committee implemented quality control procedures to verify acceptable performance of the application, to ensure that the revised baseline and sample menus met the revised meal standards, and to verify that the menus had been entered into the software application accurately.

Test Menus and Representative Baseline Menus

The committee initially wrote menus to test the practicality of possible revisions of the meal standards. To support analysis of effects of the revisions on nutrients and the possible effects of the revisions on cost, the committee identified a group of menus (called *representative baseline menus*) that provide a representation of meals currently served in the School Breakfast Program and the National School Lunch Program (NSLP).

Selection of Representative Baseline Menus SNDA-III, which includes data on the meals offered and served in a nationally representative sample of 397 schools, was the source of the menus. The committee identified menus for breakfast and lunch for each of three different school levels (elementary, middle, and high) and included equal numbers of menus planned using food-based and nutrient-based menu planning approaches. As a result of its decision to use primarily a food-based approach to menu planning, the committee identified and used a subset of six different representative baseline menu sets, each of which covered five school days. Although schools have two options for food-based menu planning (traditional or enhanced), the committee focused on traditional food-based menu planning because it is the most widely used system. About 48 percent of all schools use a traditional food-based approach, 22 percent use an enhanced food-based approach, and 30 percent use a nutrient-based approach to menu planning (USDA/FNS, 2007a). In addition, the traditional food-based menu plan requires less food than the enhanced food-based plan and thus provides a better baseline for assessing the impacts of proposed revisions on nutrient content and costs. The procedures for selecting the baseline menus appear in Appendix L.

Use of Representative Baseline and Modified Baseline Menus The committee modified the representative baseline menus as described in Chapter 6 and reviewed the results. Changes in alignment with the *Dietary Guidelines* were determined by inspection of the menus. Both the representative baseline menus and the modified baseline menus were then analyzed using the aforementioned SMMA software application. Factors considered in the analyses included changes in the nutrient content, consistency with the initial nutrient targets, and the mean cost relative to the mean cost of the representative baseline menus.

Sample Menus

Once the recommendations for the standards were finalized (see recommendations in Chapter 7), the committee wrote sample menus based on those standards, entered them in the SMMA program as described in Appendix K, and analyzed the results as described above. The sample menus appear in Appendix M, and the results of the analyses appear in Chapter 9.

DEVELOPMENT OF STANDARDS FOR MEALS *AS SELECTED* BY STUDENTS

Background

Prior to 1975, regulations for Meal Requirements were based only on meals *as offered*. At the time, a food-based menu pattern (primarily the Type A pattern mentioned in the excerpt that follows) was used as the sole approach to menu planning, and participants were required to take all five of the food components offered at lunch. In October 1975, Congress passed P.L. 94-105 (see Box 5-1), which included language targeted toward reducing food waste in the NSLP. That law led to the establishment of rules governing the number of food components that must be included in a reimbursable meal *as served*. The excerpt below summarizes the initial regulations.

> In order to ensure that children are provided as [*sic*] nutritious and well-balanced lunch, and have the opportunity to become familiar with, and enjoy different foods, present regulations require that they be served the complete lunch. In some instances this requirement has resulted in plate waste. In furtherance of the objective of reducing food waste, Pub. L. 94–105 requires that students in senior high schools participating in the National School Lunch Program not be required to accept offered foods which they do not intend to consume. The regulations have been amended so that students in senior high schools, as defined by the State and local educational agency, shall be offered all the five food items comprising the full Type A lunch and must choose at least three of these food items in order for that lunch to be eligible for Federal reimbursement. Further, the intent of Congress is reflected in the regulations to: (1) Require that if a student chooses less then [*sic*] the complete Type A lunch, the student would be expected to pay the established price of the lunch; (2) the amount of reimbursement made to any such school for such a lunch will not be affected.
>
> *Federal Register*, Vol. 41, No. 21—January 30, 1976, Proposed Rulemaking

BOX 5-1
Excerpts from Laws Relating to *Offer versus Serve*

P.L. 94-105 (October 7, 1975)
Sec. 6. Section 9 of the National School Lunch Act is amended as follows:
"(a) Subsection (a) is amended by adding at the end thereof the following new sentences: The Secretary shall establish, in cooperation with State educational agencies, administrative procedures, which shall include local educational agency and student participation, designed to diminish waste of foods which are served by schools participating in the school lunch program under this Act without endangering the nutritional integrity of the lunches served by such schools. Students in senior high schools which participate in the school lunch program under this Act shall not be required to accept offered foods which they do not intend to consume, and any such failure to accept offered foods shall not affect the full charge to the student for a lunch meeting the requirements of this subsection or the amount of payments made under this Act to any such school for such a lunch."

P.L. 95-166 (November 10, 1977)
ACCEPTANCE OF OFFERED FOODS

Sec. 8. The third sentence of section 9(a) of the National School Lunch Act is amended [by inserting the following phrase] (and, when approved by the local school district or nonprofit private schools, students in any other grade level in any junior high school or middle school).

P.L. 97-35 (August 13, 1981)
TITLE VIII—SCHOOL LUNCH AND CHILD NUTRITION PROGRAMS (95 Stat. 529)
FOOD NOT INTENDED TO BE CONSUMED

Sec. 811. The third sentence of section 9(a) of the National School Lunch Act is amended by striking out "in any junior high school or middle school."

Revised Language of the Current Law (also cited in P.L. 95-166):

Students in senior high schools that participate in the school lunch program under this Act (and, when approved by the local school district or nonprofit private schools, students in any other grade level) shall not be required to accept offered foods they do not intend to consume, and any such failure to accept offered foods shall not affect the full charge to the student for a lunch meeting the requirements of this subsection or the amount of payments made under this Act to any such school for such lunch.

P.L. 99-591 (October 30, 1986)

Sec. 331. Section 4(e) of the Child Nutrition Act of 1966 is amended by addition at the end thereof the following new paragraph: "(2) At the option of a local school food authority that participated in the school breakfast program under this Act may be allowed to refuse not more than one item of a breakfast that the student does not intend to consume. A refusal of an offered food item shall not affect the full charge to the student for a breakfast meeting the requirements of this section or the amount of payments made under this Act to a school for the breakfast."

The committee considered the relevant wording of P.L. 94-105, the excerpt of the proposed rule above, and subsequent amendments to the law (Box 5-1). Current usage refers to the *offer versus serve* (OVS) provision. OVS is mandatory for senior high schools, became optional for middle schools in 1977, and, in 1981, became optional for elementary schools as well as middle schools. The option has been adopted widely: in school year 2004–2005, SNDA-III found that 78 percent of elementary schools and 93 percent of middle schools used OVS (USDA/FNS, 2007a).

P.L. 94-105 makes it clear that the administrative procedures developed to implement the law are

1. to be established by the U.S. Department of Agriculture (the Secretary) with substantial input from state educational agencies and also with the participation of local educational agencies and students,
2. to reduce waste of foods served in the NSLP, and
3. to maintain the "nutritional integrity" of the meals served.

The current rules (typically called the *as served* meal standards) provide limits on the number (and sometimes the type) of food components that may be declined, as shown in Tables 1-1 and 1-2 in Chapter 1. These existing meal standards clearly provide a mechanism for reducing food waste. The term *as served* has been a source of confusion, however, because under OVS the food that the student is served is the food that the student selects. For this reason, the committee uses the term *standards for meals as selected* to apply to the standards for OVS. The terms *meals as served* or simply *meals served* apply to the food placed on the student's tray regardless of whether OVS is in effect.

Review of Published Evidence

A few published studies provide data relevant to setting standards for meals *as selected*. Using a visual estimation method of measuring food consumption by 457 elementary school students in Louisiana, Robichaux and Adams (1985) concluded that OVS and the traditional method of serving were generally comparable in terms of food consumption by participating students. In a study evaluating OVS at a middle-income elementary school (N = 201) and a high-poverty elementary school in Alabama (N = 170), Dillon and Lane (1989) reported the percentages of students selecting the various food components on each day of a 5-day school week. Selection of the entrée and milk approached or equaled 100 percent. Selection of a fruit serving approached 100 percent on three of the days, especially in the high-poverty school, but on one day it went as low as 44 percent in the middle-income school. The selection of grains also was high, either as part of an entrée or as an accompaniment to an entrée. In contrast, much smaller percentages of the children selected vegetables (10 to 34 percent of the children in the middle-income school and 33 to 68 percent of the children in the high-poverty school).

Analysis of data from the first School Nutrition Dietary Assessment study (SNDA-I) (USDA/FNS, 1993) revealed that NSLP participants wasted about 12 percent of the food energy and from 10 to 15 percent of the individual nutrients that they were served. The overall nutrient intakes of the students did not differ when OVS and non-OVS schools were compared. Compared with findings at non-OVS schools, smaller percentages of students of similar age were served milk at OVS schools, but they wasted less food. High school males wasted the least food (about 5 percent) and 11–14-year-old female participants wasted the most (about 17 percent).

Data from SNDA-III show that only half of the schools *served* lunches that met the existing energy standard, whereas 71 percent of the schools *offered* lunches that met the standard. Clearly, students did not select all the offered food components. Figure 5-2 allows comparison of the percentages of schools meeting existing (School Meal Initiative) standards for key nutrients *as offered* by the schools and *as served* to the students. These percentages represent averages for the schools. If a student declines food items, the nutrient content of that student's meal may be reduced substantially more than is illustrated in Figure 5-2. For example, a student who declines milk and a vegetable will have a meal that is reduced in calories, calcium, magnesium, phosphorus, zinc, vitamins A and D, B vitamins, and other nutrients.

In summary, data indicate that the use of the OVS provision has led to less waste (and therefore reduced food cost) and the selection of fewer food components by some students (therefore reduced calories and nutrients on the tray). Notably, in a multivariate analysis, predicted participation rates were significantly higher in elementary and middle schools that used OVS at lunch than in those that did not (70 percent, compared with 44 percent) (USDA/FNS, 2007a). Higher student participation rates translate to more students benefiting from school meals and more revenue for the program.

Methods

Because the standards for meals *as selected* by students apply to a large majority of elementary and middle schools as well as to all senior high schools, the committee recognized that recommendations for these standards would have a large impact on students' food selections and on the nutrient content of their meals. To provide a sound nutritional basis for the standards, the committee analyzed nutrient data related to several options for the standards at both breakfast and lunch. Then it compared

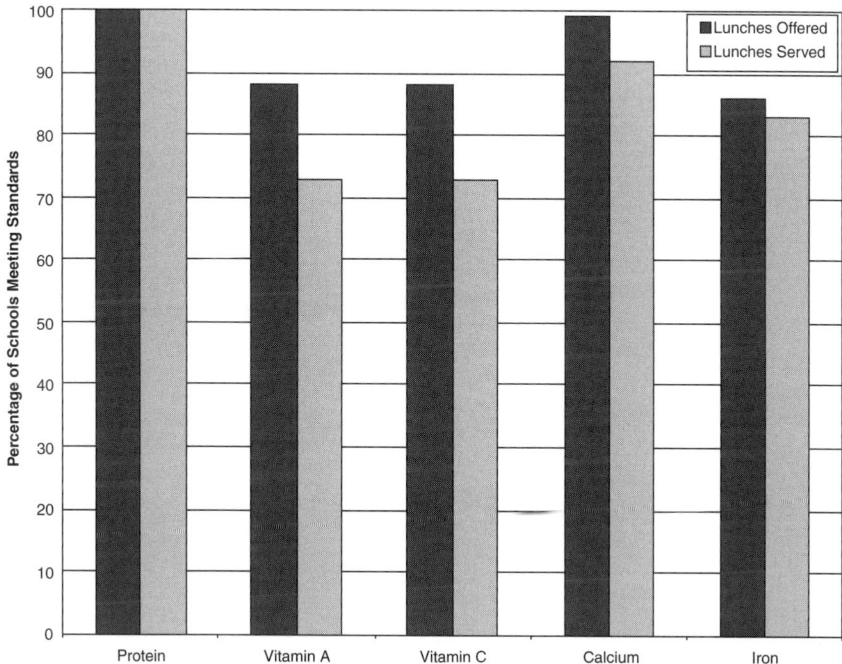

FIGURE 5-2 Percentages of schools meeting existing (School Meals Initiative) standards for key nutrients *as offered* by the schools and *as served* to the students in National School Lunch Program lunches.
SOURCE: USDA/FNS, 2007a.

estimates of the nutrient content of those options with the Nutrient Targets for the meal.

In particular, the MenuDevelopment spreadsheets were used to examine how various omissions may affect the nutrient content of school meals. The spreadsheets made it possible to estimate the effects of omitting specific types and amounts of food from the breakfast and lunch patterns for the three age-grade groups. This process provides nutrition information relevant to the specificity of the standards for meals *as selected* and to the minimum number of food items that would be allowed. The omissions that were tested appear in Box 5-2. These food items were chosen based on evidence regarding food items commonly declined by students.

Results

Tables presenting the results of the analyses appear in Appendix H (Tables H-4 through H-7). The analyses provide data on the effect of specific omissions on the approximate nutrient content of the meal (breakfast

BOX 5-2
Tests Run to Examine Effects of Omitting Food Components from the Meal Pattern

Food Items Omitted from the Breakfast Pattern	Food Items Omitted from the Lunch Pattern
• Milk • One fruit • Milk and one fruit • Two fruits	• Milk • Two vegetables • One vegetable (with different types of vegetables specified) • Milk and one vegetable (with different types of vegetables specified)

or lunch) and relate the nutrient content to the preliminary nutrient targets for the meal. The committee specifically considered nutrient shortfalls. In these summaries, the term *shortfall* applies to nutrient contents that are less than 80 percent of the Nutrient Target for the meal. As anticipated, the vitamin E content of the meals is well below the nutrient target even before testing the omission of any foods.

For breakfast, the omission of all fruit at breakfast leads to shortfalls in dietary fiber, vitamins C and B_6, magnesium, and potassium. The omission of milk at breakfast leads to different shortfalls relative to the nutrient targets for the three age-grade groups, but the vitamin D content would be very low for all. The nutrients of concern may include vitamin A, calcium, phosphorus, magnesium, and potassium, depending on the age-grade group.

The committee noted that for lunch the omission of two vegetables (that is, the case where no vegetables were selected by the student) causes the meal's content of fiber and potassium to be well under 80 percent of the Nutrient Target for all grades; magnesium would be a shortfall nutrient for high school students. Omitting milk leads to nutrient content that is well under 80 percent of the target for calcium and phosphorus, and also to shortfalls in potassium and/or riboflavin, depending on the age-grade group. In addition, the vitamin D content of the meal would be very low.

SUMMARY

This chapter describes the processes used to develop the Meal Requirements—standards for meals *as offered* by the school and *as selected* by the student. The committee used several types of analysis to inform decisions related to meal patterns and additional specifications for standards for menu planning (the *as offered* meal standards). It also used analytic methods to address the question of what and how many food items might be required for a meal to qualify for federal reimbursement under OVS (the standards for meals *as selected* by students). Chapter 6 covers some aspects of the iterative nature of the process and major challenges to the development of the Meal Requirements. Recommendations for the Meal Requirements appear in Chapter 7.

6

Iterations—Achieving the Best Balance of Nutrition, Student Acceptance, Practicality, and Cost

The development of the Nutrient Targets and Meal Requirements involved iterative processes (see Figure 2-2 in Chapter 2). The need for iteration was especially evident in the development of the recommendations for the standards for menu planning, which posed a number of major challenges. In many cases, the challenges related to the fact that menus that are based on nutrition science alone are not necessarily appealing to students, practical, or economical (or any combination of these). The challenges included finding ways to design standards for menu planning that balanced nutrition, student acceptance, practicality (including the consideration of equipment and facilities), and labor and food cost; setting the specifications for sodium; making recommendations for the definition of whole grain-rich foods; and addressing nutrient shortfalls and overages. The task of addressing standards for meals *as selected* by students under the *offer versus serve* provision of the law also posed challenges. Cost factors are addressed in Chapter 8.

NUTRIENT CONTENT, PRACTICALITY, AND APPEAL FOR THE STANDARDS OF MENU PLANNING

Amounts and types of foods specified in the initial revisions of the standards for menu planning made menu writing difficult. Challenges arose in determining the foods to include in the meat and meat alternates group; determining the amounts of certain food groups to include by meal, day, and week; and selecting acceptable forms of fluid milk. Some adjustment was needed in the calorie levels. These topics are addressed briefly below.

Foods in the Meat and Meat Alternates Group

The meat and meat alternates group in the current Meal Requirements includes all the types of food listed in MyPyramid's meat and beans group, and it also includes cheese and yogurt. MyPyramid categorizes cheese and yogurt in the milk group on the basis of nutrient content. Historically, these dairy foods have been counted as meat alternates in both school breakfast and lunch, and menu items such as a low-fat version of cheese pizza are very popular.

It quickly became evident that counting cheese and yogurt as milk substitutes rather than meat substitutes would complicate menu planning. This method would either (1) result in a decrease in the amount of fluid milk offered if cheese or yogurt was served or (2) call for an increase in milk group servings in the meal pattern so that cheese and/or yogurt could be offered along with 8 ounces of fluid milk each day. Therefore, to test the effect on nutrient intake of using cheese or yogurt as a meat substitute, the committee added lines for low-fat cheese and yogurt to the MenuDevelopment spreadsheet (see Figure 5-1 in Chapter 5). The results indicated that the content of all nutrients (except vitamin E; potassium; and, for those ages 11 years and older, iron) were above the initial targets for the meal. These three exceptions are the same nutrients that are below the targets in the pattern that includes meat. These findings support the continuation of the current practice of allowing the substitution of low-fat cheese or yogurt for meat or beans.

Determining Amounts of Food by Meal, Day, and Week

Planning daily amounts of food to meet a specific weekly pattern poses challenges, especially for the meat and meat alternates group, the grain group, and the vegetable subgroups. (See Table H-1 in Appendix H for a list of foods in the various food groups.) By testing options and examining data using the MenuDevelopment spreadsheet, it was determined that some flexibility was possible without compromising the nutritional quality of the menus. Thus, the recommended meal patterns give a range for the numbers of servings of meats and meat alternates and for the grains.

In addition, the committee determined that extra amounts of dark green or orange vegetables may be counted in the "other vegetable" subgroup. Fresh (not dried) lima beans and peas, which are both leguminous vegetables, may be counted as either a legume or a starchy vegetable. Although unsaturated vegetable oils are a MyPyramid food group, the committee determined that it was not practical to include a specified amount of oil in the recommended meal patterns for three reasons: (1) it is difficult for operators to determine the amount of vegetable oil in commercial products,

(2) school breakfast options such as cold cereal are not served with an oil, and (3) the cashier could not easily verify if a vegetable oil was on the tray. Because unsaturated vegetable oils are an important source of vitamin E, linoleic acid, and α-linolenic acid, the inclusion of unsaturated vegetable oils is encouraged within calorie limits. Maximum calorie levels were increased by 50 calories at breakfast for elementary and middle school to accommodate the changes in the recommended meal patterns.

Forms of Fluid Milk

For consistency with *Dietary Guidelines*, the committee agreed to limit the fat content of the fluid milk offered to 1 percent (the fat content of low-fat milk).[1] Knowing that *Dietary Guidelines* advises the consumption of foods and beverages with little added sugars, the committee considered advantages and disadvantages of retaining flavored milk as a milk option. The committee agreed to retain flavored fat-free milk. (Flavored low-fat milk would provide more calories and would be likely to result in menus that exceeded the calorie maximum.) Flavored milks are the predominant milk choice at school. The committee was concerned that eliminating all flavored milk would result in a substantial decrease in milk intake, especially if plain reduced-fat (2 percent milk fat) and whole milk are eliminated from the menu. Murphy and colleagues (2008) provide evidence that drinking flavored milk is positively associated with nutrient intake but not with weight status in U.S. children and adolescents. The maximum calorie level for school meals places a limit on the amount of added sugars (and solid fats) that may be included in the foods offered.

SETTING THE SPECIFICATIONS OF SODIUM

The development of standards for menu planning to meet initial sodium targets presented challenges. There are four types of major barriers to achieving substantial reductions in the sodium content of school meals:

1. *Sodium in the food supply.* The sodium content of many commercially prepared foods that are available to school meal programs is moderately high or high. For this reason, partnership by the food industry will be required to achieve substantial reductions of the sodium content of school meals. School lunches *as offered* have a mean sodium content that ranges

[1]After considering practical reasons and the nutrient content of possible meal patterns for school meals, the committee specified 1 cup of milk at both breakfast and lunch for all age-grade groups even though *Dietary Guidelines* recommends 2 rather than 3 cups of milk daily for children younger than 9 years.

from slightly less than 1,400 mg in elementary school to nearly 1,600 mg in high school (USDA/FNS, 2007a). Data from the third School Nutrition Dietary Assessment study (USDA/FNS, 2007a) also indicate that about 43 percent of the sodium in school lunches is provided by combination entrées, 17 percent by accompaniments, 12 percent by grains, and 11 percent by vegetables.

2. *Preparation of foods from ingredients that are low in salt.* If feasible, more local food preparation and the use of a greater proportion of fresh foods and frozen vegetables could result in acceptable school meals with a lower sodium content. However, many food production kitchens are designed to heat and hold food items rather than to prepare them. Additional equipment such as steamers, kettles, tilt skillets, combi ovens (combination steam and convection ovens), and perhaps refrigerators and freezers would be required to do food production. Initially, this would add to program costs. Also, switching from heat and hold to food production requires the addition of staff. Those districts that estimate meals per labor hour (MPLH) to monitor productivity may see an unfavorable decrease in their numbers.[2] Moreover, the existing kitchen facility may not be able to handle any additional equipment. This may be the case where new construction has occurred, and it also applies to older schools where space and connections of equipment may be a cost issue.

3. *Preference for salty foods.* Most schoolchildren are accustomed to the taste of salty food and tend to prefer or expect it, regardless of their participation in school meal programs. This preference or expectation is likely to persist as long as the students are routinely exposed to salty foods at home and elsewhere. There are no data to show that salt preference will decrease if the consumption of salty foods is decreased at lunch but maintained at meals outside of school.

4. *Effects on participation in school meals.* If schoolchildren are not satisfied with the taste of foods served in school meals, participation in school meal programs is likely to decrease. Children's nutrient intake and dietary quality may be reduced if they consume foods that are relatively low in nutrients and high in calories from the snack bar or vending machines or from home instead of eating the school lunch (Briefel et al., 2009; Cullen et al., 2007, 2008; Templeton et al., 2005). Children who are eligible for free or reduced-price meals may be especially vulnerable to low nutrient intake if they choose not to participate in the school meal programs. In

[2]In school food service operations, the determination of MPLH is the primary calculation used to measure labor productivity. The MPLH calculation involves equating a predetermined number of breakfast meals and snacks as well as a set dollar value of à la carte sales equal to the value of one lunch.

addition, decreased participation threatens the financial integrity of school meal programs.

These barriers are so broad in scope that school food programs, acting independently, will find it difficult to make rapid and large reductions in the sodium content of school meals. In the short term, the committee considered it unrealistic for school food authorities (SFAs) to meet the initial sodium nutrient targets from Chapter 4, which are much lower than the current amount of sodium in school meals. Nonetheless, the committee used those same values in setting sodium specifications in the standards for menu planning (see Chapter 7) but set the year 2020 as the date to achieve full implementation, with suggestions for intermediate targets.

DEFINING WHOLE GRAIN-RICH FOODS

The 2005 *Dietary Guidelines for Americans* (HHS/USDA, 2005) recommends consuming at least three 1-ounce servings of whole grains daily. It further states that, in general, half the total grain servings should be whole grains. Consequently, the standards for menu planning recommended in this report need to include specifications related to whole grains. Developing such specifications is in line with the request from the study sponsors to recommend a definition that would help schools to "easily identify whole grain products that provide a significant level of whole grains" (see Appendix C, "Critical Issues").

As a starting point, the committee noted that the grains group in MyPyramid, which is used as the basis for the meal patterns in the recommended standards for menu planning, includes two food subgroups: refined grains and whole grains. Foods in the whole grains subgroup "contain the entire grain kernel—the bran, germ, and endosperm" (USDA, 2008). Lists of whole grain ingredients appear in Appendix Table H-1 of this report and in the *HealthierUS School Challenge Whole Grains Resource Guide* (USDA/FNS, 2009b).

It is essential to distinguish between the terms *whole grains* and *whole grain-rich foods* (or *whole grain-rich products*). The term *whole grains* applies to (1) grain foods whose grain ingredients are whole grains only (100 percent whole grain, such as whole wheat bread, and oatmeal) and (2) whole grain ingredients, such as rye flour. *Whole grain-rich foods*, on the other hand, may contain less than 100 percent whole grain.

The committee recognized that it is not realistic to require that foods intended to increase the consumption of whole grains by children contain only whole grains as the grain ingredients for at least three reasons:

1. Student acceptability is very low for many foods that contain whole grains as the only grain ingredients (e.g., whole wheat bread or 100 percent whole wheat hamburger buns) (Delk and Vickers, 2007).

2. The cost of some 100 percent whole grain foods may be too high to be covered by program income.

3. The availability of whole grain food selections may be limited, especially for some small school districts.

The committee therefore focused on developing a definition of *whole grain-rich foods* that can be counted as meeting the specification for whole grains in the standards for the planning of school menus. It did so by specifying a temporary criterion that comprises two elements (one for portion size and the other for whole grain content). The criterion encompasses not only whole grains such as brown rice but also many foods that contain a mixture of whole and refined grains. (See the section "Recommended Standards for Menu Planning" in Chapter 7 for the criterion and related information.) In developing the criterion, the committee considered the strengths and limitations of various criteria that were established by different organizations (see Appendix N), while recognizing that the criterion must be relatively simple for SFAs to apply in menu planning.

In designing the meal patterns, the committee recognized that the whole grain-rich food criterion might not result in a whole grain intake that makes up half of the total grain intake (because many whole grain-rich foods are only about 50 percent whole grain). Student acceptability and cost had a major impact on the committee's recommendations related to whole grains.

MODIFYING BASELINE MENUS TO ASSESS POSSIBLE STANDARDS FOR MENU PLANNING

The committee tested the preliminary standards for menu planning in part through the process of developing *modified baseline menus*. In developing the modified menus, the objective was to retain as much of the original menu as possible, adding or substituting foods or changing portion sizes only as necessary to make the menus fit the initial menu planning standards. Based on initial attempts, minor changes were made in the standards to make the approach to menu planning more practical. The modified baseline menus were reviewed to verify improved alignment with *Dietary Guidelines*. To illustrate, Appendix L shows representative baseline menus and the corresponding modified baseline menus. Among the changes that are the easiest to notice are the types of milk (to lower fat content); substitution of whole grain-rich foods for refined grains; omission of items such as saltines and salty snacks; and substitution of lower fat meats (e.g., turkey hot dogs for regular).

To verify that the preliminary menu planning standards would lead to menus that meet or approach the preliminary nutrient targets, the committee entered the modified baseline menus into the School Meals Menu Analysis program (see Appendix K), assigned *as offered* weights for the foods using the method specified by the U.S. Department of Agriculture (USDA/FNS, 2007a), calculated the daily averages for the 5-day school week, and compared those averages to the preliminary nutrient targets. Despite the finding that the menus provided a few nutrients in amounts that were lower than the preliminary nutrient targets and that the sodium content was undesirably high (see Chapter 9), no further adjustments in either the preliminary nutrient targets or the standards for menu planning were deemed appropriate.

DETERMINATION OF STANDARDS FOR MEALS *AS SELECTED* BY STUDENTS

The law that allows students to decline some food items in school meals has two conflicting goals: decreasing waste and preserving nutritional integrity. By conducting analyses and examining the results, the committee was able to comment mainly on the nutritional aspects of options for standards for meals *as selected* by students. Because P.L. 94-102 specifies that a number of parties are to be involved in establishing the administrative procedures—that is, the standards for meals *as selected* by students—the committee considered it inappropriate to make a single recommendation for these standards. Thus, it developed two options, as discussed in Chapter 7.

SUMMARY

As guided by the experience of using the meal patterns for menu planning and the review of menus and of analyses of initial and subsequent iterations, the committee adjusted its recommended standards for menu planning as necessary to achieve a satisfactory balance of nutrition, practicality, student appeal, and cost. The initial nutrient targets were retained with the exception of calories, for which minor increases were made for some age-grade groups at breakfast. For reasons of practicality and student acceptance, the committee set a target date of the year 2020 to achieve the full implementation of the sodium specification in the meal standards but suggests the setting of intermediate targets (see Chapter 10). A temporary criterion was developed for whole grain-rich foods. Chapter 7 presents the recommendations for Nutrient Targets and Meal Requirements, and Chapter 10 covers the recommendations for bringing sodium specifications and the whole grain-rich food definition into better alignment with the *Dietary Guidelines*.

7

Recommendations for Nutrient Targets and Meal Requirements for School Meals

PRÉCIS

This chapter presents recommendations for Nutrient Targets and Meal Requirements for school meals, including explanatory information. The recommended Nutrient Targets are not intended to be used for menu planning, but they provided a basis for the development of the Meal Requirements. The Nutrient Targets differ from the existing Nutrition Standards in that they include a maximum as well as a minimum amount of calories; encompass 16 more nutrients; are higher than the current requirements for protein, vitamins A and C, calcium, and iron; and are lower than the current recommended amounts of sodium. The Nutrient Target for saturated fat is the same as in the current Nutrition Standards. To achieve agreement with *Dietary Guidelines* recommendations, however, the upper limit on total fat as a percentage of total calories was increased from 30 percent to 35 percent. Although a quantitative Nutrient Target was not set for *trans* fat, the recommended Meal Requirements include a method to keep the amount of *trans* fat in the meals as low as possible, as recommended in the *Dietary Guidelines*.

As a part of the Meal Requirements, the recommended standards for menu planning use a food-based approach that includes quantitative control of calories, saturated fat, and sodium. That is, a single set of standards is recommended for menu planning, which encompasses both food-based and nutrient-based elements. Following the standards for menu planning ensures that most of the Nutrient Targets will be met through the meals offered to the students. Exceptions are vitamin E, sometimes potassium, fats at breakfast, iron at lunch (for middle and high school levels), and sodium (because of the high sodium content of many foods). Options for standards for meals *as selected* by students are presented along with strengths and limitations of each. Options are provided because P.L. 94-105, Sec. 6(a) states that state and local educational agencies and students are to participate in the establishment of administrative procedures for reducing plate waste.

RECOMMENDED NUTRIENT TARGETS FOR THE SCHOOL BREAKFAST

Recommendation 1. The Food and Nutrition Service of the U.S. Department of Agriculture (USDA) should adopt the Nutrient Targets shown in Table 7-1 as the scientific basis for setting standards for menu planning for school meals but should not adopt a nutrient-based standard for school meal planning and monitoring.

The Nutrient Targets in Table 7-1 were developed using methods recommended by the Institute of Medicine for planning diets for groups using the Dietary Reference Intakes (IOM, 2003) and the application of the criteria in Box 2-2 of Chapter 2. Although a Nutrient Target was not set for vitamin D or *trans* fat, the standards for menu planning cover these dietary components (see later section "Recommended Meal Requirements for School Meals").

Uses of the Nutrient Targets

The main purpose for the recommended Nutrient Targets is to provide a firm scientific basis for setting standards for menu planning—that is, standards that will lead to menus that meet or nearly meet the recommended Nutrient Targets. The Nutrient Targets are not intended to be used directly for menu planning (that is, they are not intended to be used for nutrient-based menu planning). Moreover, they are not intended to be used for the monitoring of school meals (see Chapter 10). Such activities would be unrealistic in that the recommended Nutrient Targets include many nutrients for which nutrient composition data are not readily available from nutrition labels, manufacturer's specifications, or software approved by USDA for the nutrient analysis of school menus. The Nutrient Targets may be useful in evaluation and research, however.

Comparison of Recommended Targets with the Preliminary Nutrient Targets

Based on its decision regarding appropriate uses of the Nutrient Targets, the committee made no changes in the values of the preliminary nu-

TABLE 7-1 Recommended Nutrient Targets for the School Breakfast Program and the National School Lunch Program, by Meal and Age-Grade Group (Amounts per Meal Are Averages for a 5-Day School Week)

	Breakfast[a]			Lunch[b]		
Nutrient, unit	5–10 y	11–13 y	14–18 y	5–10 y	11–13 y	14–18 y
Calories (kcal)	350–500	400–550	450–600	550–650	600–700	750–850
Cholesterol (mg)*	< 65	< 65	< 65	< 96	< 96	< 96
Total Fat (% of kcal)*	25–35	25–35	25–35	25–35	25–35	25–35
Sat. Fat (% of kcal)*	<10	<10	<10	<10	<10	<10
Linoleic Acid (g)	2.2	2.5	3	3.3	3.6	4.5
α-Linolenic Acid (g)	0.21	0.25	0.3	0.31	0.36	0.45
Protein (g)	10.2	21.6	21.8	15.2	32.2	32.5
Vitamin A (μg RAE)	129	162	186	192	241	277
Vitamin C (mg)	16	20	26	24	30	39
Vitamin E (mg αT)[c]	2	2.7	3.7	3	4	5.4
Thiamin (mg)	0.2	0.3	0.4	0.4	0.5	0.6
Riboflavin (mg)	0.31	0.41	0.45	0.46	0.61	0.67
Niacin (mg)	3.2	4	4.9	4.7	6	7.3
Vitamin B_6 (mg)	0.3	0.4	0.4	0.4	0.5	0.6
Folate (μg DFE)	91	114	138	136	169	205
Vitamin B_{12} (μg)	0.8	0.9	1.1	1.2	1.3	1.6
Iron (mg)	2.3	3.5	4.0	3.4	5.2	5.9
Magnesium (mg)	49	66	99	72	98	147
Zinc (mg)	2	2.5	2.9	2.9	3.7	4.3
Calcium (mg)	223	296	323	332	440	481
Phosphorus (mg)	242	362	384	361	538	572
Potassium (mg)[c]	909	1,023	1,169	1,353	1,523	1,740
Sodium (mg)[d]	≤ 434	≤ 473	≤ 495	≤ 636	≤ 704	≤ 736
Fiber (g)	5.7	6.3	7.2	8.5	9.4	10.7

NOTES: αT = α-tocopherol; DFE = dietary folate equivalents; g = gram; kcal = calories; kg = kilogram; mg = milligrams; RAE = retinol activity equivalents; Sat. = saturated; μg = micrograms; y = years.

[a]Targets based on 21.5 percent of the daily School Meal-Target Median Intake for the age-grade group.

[b]Targets based on 32 percent of the daily School Meal-Target Median Intake for the age-grade group.

[c]Targets for vitamin E and potassium are known to be higher than can be expected following meal plans based on MyPyramid.

[d]Targets for sodium, which are based on the Tolerable Upper Intake Level, are for the year 2020.

SOURCE: *HHS/USDA, 2005.

trient targets other than to increase the maximum calorie level for two of the grade groups at breakfast (see Chapter 6). That is, the recommended Nutrient Targets are essentially the same as the preliminary nutrient targets that are discussed in Chapter 4.

In those cases in which it is very difficult to meet the Nutrient Targets, which are based largely on the Dietary Reference Intakes, the values can serve as goals. For example, school meal programs could be encouraged to incorporate rich sources of vitamin E and potassium in their menus more often, to reduce the amount of sodium in the foods that are offered, and to increase the use of vegetable oils or soft margarine at breakfast (within calorie limits).

Comparison of the Recommended Nutrient Targets with Existing Nutrition Standards for the School Meal Programs

Comparison with the existing Nutrition Standards is not straightforward because the recommended age-grade ranges differ from the existing ranges. Appendix O presents the data for calories and the nutrients that are common to both the standards and the targets, and it lists the additional nutrients contained in the recommended targets. Notably, compared to the current Nutrition Standards, the recommended Nutrient Targets are higher for protein and the vitamins and minerals, the recommended minimum calorie levels are lower, and maximum calorie levels have been set for the first time. The maximum calorie levels are similar, and in some cases lower, than the existing minimum calorie standards.

Comparison of Possible Nutrient Targets Derived Using Different Methods

Because the recommendations for Nutrient Targets were developed using methods that differ from those set out in P.L. 104-193 (1)(B), it is essential to compare the recommended Nutrient Targets with values that would have been developed using the previously accepted method, which was based on using specified fractions of the Recommended Dietary Allowances (RDAs) of the Food and Nutrition Board. The committee compared all the recommended Nutrient Targets for protein, vitamins, and minerals with the values it calculated for the same nutrients using the most recent RDAs or Adequate Intakes (AIs) as the reference standard.[1] Table 7-2 shows the comparisons for the high school age-grade group (ages 14–18 years, grades 9–11). Tables for elementary school and middle school may be found in Appendix O.

All the recommended Nutrient Targets are higher than those that would have been set using the current RDAs or AIs, with one or two exceptions. The recommended standard for α-linolenic acid is very slightly lower than that based on the AI for ages 5–10 years, and the recommended standard for linoleic acid for the children ages 5–10 years is the same as the AI. The Nutrient Targets have higher values as a result of the committee's

[1]The comparison excludes sodium. For sodium, the objective is to reduce the amount rather than to be sure to provide enough.

TABLE 7-2 Comparison of the Recommended Nutrient Targets for the School Breakfast Program and the National School Lunch Program with Values Based on the Recommended Dietary Allowances or Adequate Intake, High School (Ages 14 Through 18 Years)

			Breakfast Targets[a]		Lunch Targets[b]	
Nutrient	SM-TMI	Current RDA/AI	Nutrient Targets	RDA/AI Method	Nutrient Targets	RDA/AI Method
Protein (g)	101.6	49	21.8	12.3	32.5	16.3
Vitamin A (μg RAE)[c]	867	800	186	200	277	266
Vitamin C (mg)[c]	121	70	26	18	39	23
Vitamin E (mg αT)	17	15	3.7	3.8	5.4	5.0
Thiamin (mg)[c]	1.74	1.1	0.37	0.28	0.56	0.37
Riboflavin (mg)[c]	2.08	1.2	0.45	0.29	0.67	0.38
Niacin (mg)[c]	22.7	15	4.9	3.8	7.3	5.0
Vitamin B_6 (mg)	1.97	1.3	0.42	0.33	0.63	0.43
Folate (μg DFE)	640	400	138	100	205	133
Vitamin B_{12} (μg)	5.1	2.4	1.1	0.6	1.6	0.8
Iron (mg)[c]	18.4	13.0	4.0	3.3	5.9	4.3
Magnesium (mg)[c]	459	385	99	96	147	128
Zinc (mg)[c]	13.5	10.0	2.9	2.5	4.3	3.2
Calcium (mg)	1,504	*1,300*	323	325	481	416
Phosphorus (mg)	1,787	1,250	384	313	572	400
Potassium (mg)	5,438	*4,700*	1,169	1,175	1,740	1,504
Sodium (mg)	2,300[d]	*1,500*	≤ 495[d]	375[e]	≤ 736[d]	480[e]
Linoleic Acid (g)	14.1	*13.5*	3.0	3.4	4.5	4.3
α-Linolenic Acid (g)	1.41	*1.4*	0.30	0.34	0.45	0.43
Fiber (g)[c]	33.5	*32.0*	7.2	8.0	10.7	10.7

NOTES: AIs are presented in italics. AI = Adequate Intake; αT = α-tocopherol; d = day; DFE = dietary folate equivalent; g = gram; kg = kilogram; mg = milligram; RAE = retinol activity equivalents; RDA = Recommended Dietary Allowance; SM-TMI = School Meal-Target Median Intake; μg = microgram; y = years.

[a]Nutrient Targets based on 21.5 percent of the School Meal-TMI; RDA/AI Method values are based on 25 percent of the RDA or AI.

[b]Nutrient Targets based on 32 percent of the School Meal-TMI; RDA/AI Method values are based on 33.3 percent of the RDA or AI.

[c]RDA/AI expressed as mean for males and females.

[d]Targets for sodium, which are based on the Tolerable Upper Intake Level, are for the year 2020.

[e]Values for sodium are based on the AI for sodium

SOURCE: *IOM, 2006.

intent to reduce the prevalence of inadequate intakes of nutrients[2] among schoolchildren (Criterion 1 in Box 2-2) rather than simply ensure that the mean intake equals the RDA.[3] In choosing Nutrient Targets that are high

[2]That is, a low prevalence of intakes below the Estimated Average Requirement.

[3]Although intake at the RDA should result in a low probability of inadequacy for a given individual, mean intake at the RDA for a group of people does not usually result in a low

enough to result in a low predicted prevalence of nutrient inadequacy, the committee recognizes that the nutrient density (nutrients per 100 calories) of the school meals will need to increase. School meals with an increased nutrient density will hopefully serve as a model for meals and snacks that children consume outside the school setting and will result in improvements of their total day's diet.

Thus, with the above-noted minor exceptions, the recommended Nutrient Targets are consistent with P.L. 104-193, which states that the school meals must provide *at least* one-third of the RDA for lunch and *at least* one-fourth of the RDA for breakfast. With respect to calories, the recommended Nutrient Targets are consistent with P.L. 104-193 in that they "are consistent with the goals of the most recent Dietary Guidelines for Americans" (namely, adequate nutrients within energy needs [HHS/USDA, 2005]), and the RDAs do not apply to calories. Importantly, however, to be consistent with *Dietary Guidelines*, the recommended standards for menu planning are primarily derived from the MyPyramid food patterns, rather than from the Nutrient Targets. As noted in Chapters 4 and 5, the nutrient values of the MyPyramid food patterns are almost always higher than the School Meal-Target Median Intake values that were the basis of the Nutrient Targets for school meals.

Sodium is a special case in that (1) the *Dietary Guidelines* calls for reduced intake and (2) the recommended Nutrient Targets are based on the Tolerable Upper Intake Levels (ULs) for the age-grade groups rather than on the AI. The recommended Nutrient Targets for sodium are slightly lower than the values that would correspond to the *Dietary Guidelines* recommendation because the ULs are lower for children and adolescents.

RECOMMENDED MEAL REQUIREMENTS FOR SCHOOL MEALS

Meal Requirements encompass (1) the standards for menu planning, which apply to the foods that are prepared and set out for the students and (2) the standards for meals *as selected* by the student, which apply to the foods the student has on his or her tray, as checked by the cashier. The recommended Meal Requirements are intended for all school food service

---

prevalence of inadequacy for the group. Because the person-to-person variation in intake is very high within a group, it is almost always necessary to aim for a group mean intake above the RDA to ensure a low prevalence of inadequacy. For this reason, the method the committee used to set the School Meal-Target Median Intakes results in values that are uniformly above the RDA, and the breakfast and lunch Nutrient Targets are correspondingly higher than targets that would result from an approach that was based on having the group mean equal to the RDA. For nutrients with either an AI or an RDA, the use of the nutrient density approach rather than the use of the average Target Median Intake (as described in Chapter 4) also resulted in higher Nutrient Targets for some nutrients.

operations, regardless of the approach to menu planning that is currently in use.

Recommended Standards for Menu Planning

Based on the results of the committee's analysis of test meal patterns and menus, the information presented in Chapter 6 on challenges, and consideration of the committee's four criteria set out in Chapter 2, the committee developed a single set of standards for menu planning.

> **Recommendation 2. To align school meals with the *Dietary Guidelines for Americans* and improve the healthfulness of school meals, the Food and Nutrition Service should adopt standards for menu planning that increase the amounts of fruits, vegetables and whole grains; increase the focus on reducing the amounts of saturated fat and sodium provided; and set a minimum and maximum level of calories—as presented in Table 7-3.**

The standards depicted in Table 7-3 include elements from three existing USDA meal planning approaches—namely, the traditional food-based, enhanced food-based, and nutrient-based menu planning approaches. In particular, the standards for menu planning include

- food-based meal patterns that cover the types and amounts of food groups and subgroups to be offered by age-grade group;
- specifications for minimum and maximum calorie levels and for the maximum level of saturated fat;
- specifications for sodium that are to be attained by the year 2020, with suggestions for intermediate targets (see Chapter 10); and
- specifications for *trans* fat that limit the amount of *trans* fat that any commercial food product may contain.

As explained in the section "Consideration of Meal Planning Approaches" in Chapter 5, the committee did not develop standards for a nutrient-based menu planning approach. The committee's recommended standards for menu planning do not preclude the use of a comprehensive nutrient analysis in menu planning if an operator wants to compare the nutrient content of the menus with the Nutrient Targets, but nutrient analysis software to accomplish this task for all the Nutrient Targets is not currently available. Nonetheless, existing USDA-approved nutrient analysis software can simplify the process of implementing the committee's recommended standards for menu planning. In particular, the software can help in choosing items from food groups that will keep the calorie and saturated

TABLE 7-3 Recommended *as Offered* Meal Standards

	Breakfast			Lunch		
	Grades K–5	Grades 6–8	Grades 9–12	Grades K–5	Grades 6–8	Grades 9–12
Meal Pattern	Amount of Foods[a] Per Week					
Fruits (cups)[b]	5	5	5	2.5	2.5	5
Vegetables (cups)[b]	0	0	0	3.75	3.75	5
Dark green	0	0	0	0.5[c]	0.5[c]	0.5[c]
Orange	0	0	0	0.5[c]	0.5[c]	0.5[c]
Legumes	0	0	0	0.5[c]	0.5[c]	0.5[c]
Starchy	0	0	0	1	1	1
Other	0	0	0	1.25[c]	1.25[c]	2.5[c]
Grains, at least half of which must be whole grain-rich[d] (oz eq)	7–10	8–10	9–10	9–10	9–10	12–13
Meats, beans, cheese, yogurt (oz eq)	5	5	7–10	8–10	9–10	10–12
Fat-free milk (plain or flavored) or low-fat milk (1% milk fat or less) (cups)	5	5	5	5	5	5
Other Specifications	Other Specifications: Daily Amount Based on the Average for a 5-Day Week					
Min-max calories (kcal)[e,f]	350–500	400–550	450–600	550–650	600–700	750–850
Saturated fat (% of total calories)[g]	< 10	< 10	< 10	< 10	< 10	< 10
Sodium (mg)	[≤ 430]	[≤ 470]	[≤ 500]	[≤ 640]	[≤ 710]	[≤ 740]
	Sodium targets are to be reached by the year 2020.[h]					
trans fat	Nutrition label must specify zero grams of *trans* fat per serving.[i]					

NOTES: K = kindergarten; kcal = calories; max = maximum; mg = milligrams; min = minimum; oz eq = ounce equivalent. Although the recommended weekly meal intake patterns do not specify amounts of unsaturated oils, their use is to be encouraged within calorie limits.

[a]Food items included in each group and subgroup and amount equivalents. Appendix Table H-1 gives a listing of foods by food group and subgroup. Minimum daily requirements apply: 1/5 of the weekly requirement for fruits, total vegetables, and milk and at least 1oz equivalent each of grains and meat or meat alternate (2 oz of each for grades 9–12 lunch).

[b]One cup of fruits and vegetables usually provides two servings; ¼ cup of dried fruit counts as ½ cup of fruit; 1 cup of leafy greens counts as ½ cup of vegetables. No more than half of the fruit offerings may be in the form of juice.

[c]Larger amounts of these vegetables may be served.

[d]Based on at least half of the grain content as whole grain. Aiming for a higher proportion of whole grain-rich foods is encouraged. See Box 7-1 for Temporary Criterion for Whole-Grain Rich Foods. Also note that in Chapter 10 the committee recommends that the Food Buying Guide serving sizes be updated to be consistent with MyPyramid Equivalent serving sizes.

[e]The average daily amount for a 5-day school week is not to be less than the minimum or exceed the maximum.

[f]Discretionary sources of calories (for example, solid fats and added sugars) may be added to the meal pattern if within the specifications for calories, saturated fat, *trans* fat, and sodium.

[g]The average daily amount for a 5-day school week is not to exceed the maximum.

[h]To ensure that action is taken to reduce the sodium content of school meals over the 10-year period in a manner that maintains student participation rates, the committee suggests the setting of intermediate targets for each 2-year interval. (See the section "Achieving Long-Term Goals" in Chapter 10.)

[i]Because the nutrition facts panel is not required for foods with Child Nutrition labeling, the committee suggests that only products with 0 grams of *trans* fat per serving be eligible for consideration for such labeling.

fat levels within the calorie and saturated fat specifications in Table 7-3 and help monitor progress on reducing the sodium content of meals. Moreover, computerized nutrient analysis may be helpful to parents of schoolchildren with special dietary needs. Computerized nutrient analysis is not essential, however, as long as operators use an accepted method to control the calorie, saturated fat, and sodium content of school meals.

Food-based Meal Patterns

Dietary Guidelines for Americans (HHS/USDA, 2005) emphasizes the use of foods to meet nutrient needs:

> A basic premise of the *Dietary Guidelines* is that nutrient needs should be met primarily through consuming foods. Foods provide an array of nutrients (as well as phytochemicals, antioxidants, etc.) and other compounds that may have beneficial effects on health.
>
> HHS/USDA, 2005, p. 3

The food-based meal patterns shown in Table 7-3 were designed to be consistent with *Dietary Guidelines* and to be consistent with the recommended Nutrient Targets by age-grade group. Menus written to correspond with the meal patterns shown in Table 7-3 were demonstrated, through the use of nutrient analysis, to meet or nearly meet the standards for protein, vitamins, minerals, and other dietary components like fatty acids, with a few exceptions. The fluid milk that is specified in the standards for menu planning provides one-half of the AI for vitamin D at each school meal.

Specifications for Calories, Saturated Fat, and Sodium

The use of meal patterns alone cannot ensure that calories, saturated fat, and sodium are consistent with *Dietary Guidelines*. Because of this, the recommended standards for menu planning include specifications for calories, saturated fat, and sodium, with the understanding that the sodium specification is to be achieved by the year 2020 (see Chapter 10).

Operators will need to use some quantitative method to ensure that, on average for the 5-day school week, the menus provide calories within the specified limits and less than 10 percent of the calories from saturated fat (a possible approach is given in Chapter 10); and they will need to monitor their progress in reducing the average daily sodium content of the school meals.

Forms of Food for School Meals

The meal patterns were designed assuming that the following forms of food would be used in planning menus:

- Fruits will be fresh, frozen without sugar, dried, or canned in fruit juice, water, or light syrup.
- If canned vegetables are purchased, they will contain no added salt or will be reduced in sodium content.
- To be classified as a whole grain-rich food as part of the meal standards, the food will meet the whole grain-rich food criterion shown in Box 7-1.

BOX 7-1
Temporary Criterion for Whole Grain-Rich Foods

Both elements of the criterion must be met for a food to qualify as a whole grain-rich food:

Element #1. A serving of the food item must be at least the portion size of one Grains/Breads serving as defined in the *USDA Food Buying Guide for Child Nutrition Programs* (USDA/FNS, 2009c).

AND

Element #2. The food must meet at least *one* of the following:

a. The whole grains* per serving (based on minimum serving sizes specified for grains/breads in the *USDA Food Buying Guide for Child Nutrition Programs*) (USDA/FNS, 2009c) must be ≥ 8 grams. This may be determined from information provided on the product packaging or by the manufacturer, if available.
b. The product includes the following Food and Drug Administration (FDA)-approved whole grain health claim on its packaging. "Diets rich in whole grain foods and other plant foods, and low in saturated fat and cholesterol may help reduce the risk of heart disease."
c. Product ingredient listing lists whole grain first, specifically,
   I. *Non-mixed dishes (e.g., breads, cereals):* Whole grains must be the primary ingredient by weight (a whole grain is the first ingredient in the list)
   II. *Mixed dishes (e.g., pizza, corn dogs):* Whole grains must be the primary grain ingredient by weight (a whole grain is the first grain ingredient in the list)

   For foods prepared by the school food service, the recipe is used as the basis for a calculation to determine whether the total weight of whole grain ingredients exceeds the total weight of non-whole grain ingredients. Detailed instructions for this method appear in the *HealthierUS School Challenge Whole Grains Resource* guide (USDA/FNS, 2009b).

---

*Whole grain ingredients are those specified in the *HealthierUS School Challenge Whole Grain Resource* guide (www.fns.usda.gov/TN/HealthierUS/wholegrainresource.pdf).

- Meats will be lean. Soy extenders are acceptable. Although meats that are preserved by smoking, curing, or salting, or by the addition of preservatives are sometimes lean, they usually are very high in sodium. Because of their sodium content and because the consumption of such processed meats, especially processed red meats, has been linked with an increased risk of colorectal cancer in adults (WCRF/AICR, 2007), less frequent use of even low-fat versions of these meats may be advisable.
- Cheese and yogurt will be low fat.
- Milk offerings will be fat-free (plain or flavored) or low-fat (1 percent milk fat or less, plain only).
- Foods (such as salad dressing, dips, muffins, some entrées, and some vegetable dishes) that contain added "fat" will be made with unsaturated oils. The use of some unsaturated oils is encouraged because they provide vitamin E and essential fatty acids.
- If purchased commercially, the nutrition labeling or manufacturer's specification will indicate that the product contains 0 g of *trans* fat per serving.

Guidance for reducing sodium in school meals may be obtained from several resources, including http://teamnutrition.usda.gov/Resources/DGfact sheet_sodium.pdf and the SMI Road to Success booklet (USDA/FNS, 2007b).

The recommended temporary criterion for whole grain-rich foods (Box 7-1) merits special attention. It is based in large part on what is currently possible considering that current labeling regulations and practices limit the school food service purchaser's ability to know the actual whole grain content of many grain products. Although the goal of the criterion is to ensure that foods qualify as whole grain-rich if they contain at least 8 g of whole grains, some foods with lower amounts of whole grains may be classified as whole grain rich if the product ingredient listing (item c under element #2 of the criterion) is used as one of the indicators of whole grain content.

At this time, product ingredient listing is an essential element of the temporary criterion for two reasons: (1) manufacturers are not required to provide information about the grams of whole grains in their products, and many do not provide that information; and (2) the FDA whole grain health claim is not mandatory. Rather, manufacturers are allowed to place this claim on product packaging if whole grain, fat, fatty acid, and cholesterol content requirements for this health claim are met.

It is important to note that whole grain foods (such as brown rice) and some other foods that contain substantially more than 8 g of whole grain per grain serving may be classified as whole grain rich using the temporary criterion. Consequently, although some foods with less than 8 grams of whole grain may count as whole grain-rich, so too will some foods with substantially more than 8 g of whole grain per 1 ounce equivalent serving.

The committee views the criterion for whole grain-rich foods included in this report as temporary. Recommendations to improve the criterion in coming years appear in Chapter 10.

Standards for Menu Planning for Different Grade Configurations

The standards in Table 7-3 make allowance for a number of possible grade configurations in schools. For example, the same general meal pattern could be used for students from kindergarten through grade 8. In those instances where the grade configuration differs, as in schools that serve elementary through high school students on the same line, the committee suggests that the school food authority work with the state agency to find a solution that ensures that the basic elements of the standards for menu planning will be maintained: inclusion of the specified food groups and food subgroups, moderate calorie values, and an emphasis on reducing saturated fat and sodium.

Recommended Standards for Menu Planning and the Current Law

The *Healthy Meals for Children Act of 1996* (P.L. 104-149, Sec. 2) increased the flexibility of schools to meet the *Dietary Guidelines for Americans* under the National School Lunch Act. In particular, it amends that act to allow the use of any reasonable approach, within guidelines established by the Secretary of Agriculture, but "The Secretary may not require a school to conduct or use a nutrient analysis to meet the requirements of this paragraph." The recommended standards for menu planning could be implemented under this law.

The committee's recommendation calls for only one approach to menu planning—an approach that is based primarily on foods and entails that quantitative attention be given only to the calorie, saturated fat, and sodium content of the meal. A food-based approach is the only dependable approach to meeting most of the *Dietary Guidelines*. However, the committee's experience in developing an approach to menu planning (and the evidence presented in the third School Nutrition Dietary Assessment study [SNDA-III] report) has shown that it is difficult to control the calorie, saturated fat, and sodium content of menus without using quantitative methods that ordinarily come under the category of "nutrient analysis." Notably, the sponsor requested that the committee "examine the adequacy of the current menu planning approaches in meeting the applicable [Dietary Reference Intakes] and [*Dietary Guidelines for Americans*]" and expressed concern that the current menu planning approaches . . . may no longer be adequate to provide school meals that reflect the 2005 [*Dietary Guidelines for Americans*]" (see Appendix C). The recommended standards for menu planning provide an approach that removes that concern.

Compared with the recommended standards for menu planning, a somewhat less specific set of standards (one without the quantitative component) could help move school meal programs in the direction of meeting the recommended Nutrient Targets and the *Dietary Guidelines*, but only partway. The recommended standards are presented as the most nutritionally sound yet practical approach to planning menus that will appeal to schoolchildren.

Options for Standards for Meals *as Selected* by Students

Under the *offer versus serve* (OVS) provision of P.L. 94-105, all high schools must allow students to select a smaller number of food items than are offered at lunch. OVS is optional at breakfast for all the grades, and it is optional for lunch in elementary and middle schools. The current standards specify the number of food components and sometimes a type of food component that must be on a student's tray if the meal is to be reimbursable.

Recommendation 3. To achieve a reasonable balance between the goals of reducing waste and preserving the nutritional integrity of school meals, the Food and Nutrition Service, in conjunction with state and local educational agencies and students, should weigh the strengths and limitations of the committee's two options (see Table 7-4) when setting standards for the meals *as selected* by students.

Based on its reading of the OVS provision of P.L. 94-105 and the committee's consideration of nutrition, practicality, and cost, the committee decided that the most useful course of action would be to put forth two options for standards for meals *as selected* by the student (Table 7-4). Option 1, the committee's preferred option, is similar to the current standard, but it offers the advantage of encouraging the consumption of fruits and vegetables, in line with the *Dietary Guidelines for Americans*. The student would be able to select from at least two fruit or vegetable items. Option 2 allows the student to decline an additional food item and thus may decrease waste, but the nutritional integrity of the meal would be lower (see Tables H-4 through H-7 in Appendix H). The committee notes that option 2 for breakfast is inconsistent with Amendments to the *National School Lunch Act* and *Child Nutrition Act* (1986), Sec. 331 Extension of Offer Versus Serve Provision to the School Breakfast Program, Section 4(e) of the *Child Nutrition Act of 1966* (42 U.S.C. 1773(e)), which states that students may

TABLE 7-4 Options for Standards for Meals *as Selected* by the Student under the *Offer Versus Serve* Provision of P.L. 94-105[a]

	Number of Items the Student May Decline and Required Items	
	Breakfast	Lunch
1. Preferred	One item[b] may be declined, must take at least one fruit or juice	Two items may be declined, must take at least one fruit or vegetable
2. Alternative	Two items may be declined, must take at least one fruit or juice	Three items may be declined, must take at least one fruit or vegetable

NOTE: Options are provided for consideration by the U.S. Department of Agriculture, working cooperatively with state educational agencies and with participation by local educational agencies and student to develop new regulations. The committee recommends Option 1.

[a]Under current traditional food-based menu planning standards, high school students are required to take three out of four (or five) food items at breakfast and three out of five food items at lunch. *Offer versus serve* is optional for elementary and middle schools.

[b]A specific food offered in the specified portion sizes that will meet the recommended *as offered* Meal Requirements.

decline no more than one item at breakfast. Because the number of items has been increased in the recommended standards for menu planning, however, allowing students to decline two items could be a reasonable approach for breakfast. At either breakfast or lunch, option 2 (which would allow the student to select fewer food items) may be more appropriate for high school females who have low energy needs. These options provide those involved in establishing administrative procedures (USDA, with input from state and local educational agencies and students) with information that may guide their decision-making process. The committee's considerations in developing options are summarized briefly below.

Nutritional Considerations

There is concern that OVS will result in lower nutrient intake at school breakfast and lunch because children are allowed to decline items, especially if they decline the most nutrient-rich food components (e.g., fruits, vegetables, whole grain-rich foods, milk). Appendix H gives examples of how declining specific food components affect the average nutrient content of the meal. The omission of milk, in particular, substantially reduces the content of calcium, magnesium, potassium, and many vitamins and other nutrients. However, this concern about OVS would be valid only if children would indeed eat all of the food components included in the standard meal plan if served. Because child taste and food preferences and state of hunger and satiety play strong roles in regulating food consumption, for some children the food and nutrient content of a school meal *as offered* by the school will exceed the child's food and nutrient intake from that meal, regardless of the OVS regulations that are in place.

Assuming wise food choices by the student, the least amount of restriction of choice might provide a nutritional advantage for children whose energy needs are lower than the levels targeted by the standard meal pattern. Theoretically, the second option, which is less restrictive, would provide children the opportunity to better match their meal selection with individual energy needs. Although option 1 (which allows the student to decline fewer items) would result in more food on the student's tray, it would not necessarily result in the consumption of more foods.

Practical Considerations

The options presented by the committee were influenced by practical considerations relating to the cafeteria setting. The typical cafeteria moves 7 to 10 students through the line per minute, and the flow in some cafeterias may exceed 14 students per minute through the line. The student is making quick food selections, often with little prior contemplation other than on the entrée selection (if a choice is offered and was publicized), while little thought is given to the other choices. The cashier is responsible for recording the meal sale (which may involve ticket collection, roster checklist, accepting the meal identification card, or key pad entry into the point-of-sale software system), often taking cash and checks and making change, and verifying whether the meal on the tray meets the requirements for meals *as selected* by the student. If the meal does not meet the requirements, the meal will not be reimbursable unless the student takes something additional from the line. Although there may be creative ways of facilitating that, the line is likely to be slowed somewhat. Thus, to ensure that the OVS provisions will be followed, the standard for meals *as selected* by the student must be easy for students and staff to follow. The committee's two options were selected with that objective in mind.

Cost Considerations

Giving choices helps to reduce waste and thus cost for the overall program. For this reason, although options 1 and 2 both list a specific food requirement, the requirement allows choice among two or more foods. If an option required a vegetable, a vegetable would be selected but might not be eaten. An option to require a serving of fluid milk was ruled out because milk intolerance or avoidance is relatively common among some racial, ethnic, and religious groups, and some children will not drink the lower fat varieties of milk until they are more familiar with them. If the child does not consume the food, requiring a vegetable or milk leads to waste rather than improved nutrient intake.

SUMMARY

The recommended Nutrient Targets provide a scientific underpinning for the Meal Requirements, but the targets are not meant for menu planning. The Nutrient Targets differ from the existing Nutrition Standards in that they include a maximum as well as a minimum level of calories; encompass 16 additional nutrients; are higher for the 8 nutrients that are common to both; and, for most nutrients, are based on a Target Median Intake rather than the Recommended Dietary Allowances. Under the Meal Requirements, the recommended standards for menu planning provide a food-based approach that encompasses five major food groups and seven food subgroups; it also provides specifications for calories, saturated fat, and sodium; a method to minimize *trans* fat content, and a temporary criterion to identify whole grain-rich foods. The options presented for standards for meals *as selected* by the student are accompanied by information on nutrition-related strengths and concerns of each option.

8

Food Cost Implications and Market Effects

This chapter provides a description of methods and results of the committee's analysis of the food cost implications of the recommended changes to the Meal Requirements. The effects of proposed changes in the market are also considered.

CHANGES IN AMOUNTS AND TYPES OF FOOD

A change in the Meal Requirements could have a major effect on the cost of food to School Food Authorities (SFAs) if there are large changes in the types and amounts of foods required by the standards for menu planning and the standards for meals *as selected*. Tables 8-1 and 8-2 show that there are substantial differences in the amounts and types of foods specified in the current and recommended standards for menu planning, especially with regard to fruits, vegetables, and whole grain-rich foods. The main difference in the current and recommended standards for meals *as selected* is the new recommendation that students select at least one fruit at breakfast and at least one fruit or vegetable at lunch. In addition, the recommended requirements effectively increase the recommended amounts of meat or meat alternate, especially for the elementary level. Many other factors also affect the cost and sources of foods in school meal programs. It was not possible for the committee to address all these factors in its analyses to evaluate the food costs, but relevant factors are discussed in the later section "Other Factors Affecting Meal Costs."

TABLE 8-1 School Breakfast Program: Current Requirements Compared to Recommendations for a 5-Day School Week[a]

	Current Requirements	Recommendations		
Grade Levels	K–12	K–5	6–8	9–12
Fruit (cups)	2.5	5	5	5
Vegetable (cups)	0	0	0	0
Grain/Bread (oz eq)	0–10[b,c]	7–10[d]	8–10[d]	9–10[d]
Meat/Meat Alternates (oz eq)	0–10[c]	5	5	7–10
Milk (cups)	5	5	5	5

NOTE: oz eq = ounce equivalent.

[a]Requirements and recommendations are for meals *as offered* for a 5-day school week. Requirements are minimum portion sizes based on the Traditional Food-Based Menu planning approach.

[b]Must be enriched or whole grain.

[c]Requirements call for two grains, two meats, or one of each.

[d]At least half of which must be whole grain-rich (i.e., meet the criterion in Box 7-1).

SOURCE: USDA/FNS, 2008e.

METHODS USED TO EVALUATE COSTS AND CHANGES IN THE COST OF FOOD FOR REPRESENTATIVE BASELINE SCHOOL MENUS

Assessing the impact of changes to the Meal Requirements on the food costs of reimbursable[1] breakfast and reimbursable lunch meals requires data on (1) the changes in the amounts and types of foods used when a representative (typical or average) meal is compared with the same meal modified to meet the Meal Requirements and (2) the prices of the individual food items used in each meal.

Data from recent, nationally representative school surveys were used in establishing the representative baseline menus and the food costs used in this report. In overview, the committee

1. Selected a set of 12 representative baseline menus (each of which covered 5 school days) for the breakfast and lunch meals, drawing from menus available in the third School Nutrition Dietary Assessment study (SNDA-III) data, as described and illustrated in Chapter 6. The complete set of baseline menus included five school-day menus from each age-grade level for each of the two meals and for the two major menu-planning approaches (food- and nutrient-based);

[1]Reimbursable meals are meals that meet the requirements outlined in the section "School Meals Program Overview" in Chapter 1.

TABLE 8-2 School Lunch Program: Current Requirements Compared to Recommendations for a 5-Day School Week[a]

	Current Requirements: Traditional Food-Based Approach			Current Requirements: Enhanced Food-Based Approach			Recommendations		
Grade Levels	K–3[b]	4–12[b]	7–12[c,d]	K–3[b,d]	K–6[b]	7–12	K–5	6–8	9–12
Fruit (cups)	2.5[e]	3.75[e]	3.75[e]	3.75[e]	4.25[g]	5[e]	2.5	2.5	5
Vegetable (cups)							3.75	3.75	5
Dark Green	NS	NS	NS	NS	NS	NS	0.5	0.5	0.5
Orange	NS	NS	NS	NS	NS	NS	0.5	0.5	0.5
Legumes	NS	NS	NS	NS	NS	NS	0.5	0.5	0.5
Starchy	NS	NS	NS	NS	NS	NS	1	1	1
Other	NS	NS	NS	NS	NS	NS	1.25	1.25	2.5
Grain/Bread (oz eq)	8 (min 1/day)[f]	8 (min 1/day)[f]	10 (min 1/day)[f]	10 (min 1/day)[f]	12 (min 1/day)[f]	15 (min 1/day)[f]	9–10[h]	9–10[h]	12–13[h]
Meat/Meat Alternates (oz eq)	7.5	10	15	7.5	10	10	8–10	9–10	10–12
Milk (cups)	5	5	5	5	5	5	5	5	5

NOTES: min = minimum; NS = not specified; oz eq = ounce equivalents.

[a]Requirements and recommendations are for meals *as offered* for a 5-day school week.

[b]Minimum portion sizes.

[c]Recommended portion sizes under the Traditional Food-Based Menu planning approach.

[d]Optional grade configuration.

[e]Two or more servings of fruit, vegetables, or both a day.

[f]Must be enriched or whole grain.

[g]Two or more servings of fruit, vegetables, or both a day, plus an extra half-cup over the 5-day school week.

[h]At least half of which must be whole grain-rich (i.e., meet the criteria in Box 7-1).

SOURCE: USDA/FNS, 2000a.

2. Matched food items in the 2004–2005 menus (from the school year when the SNDA-III data were collected) to food codes in cost data collected during school year 2005–2006 through the School Lunch and Breakfast Cost Study (SLBCS)-II (USDA/FNS, 2008f) and supplemented the cost data as described below;

3. Estimated the cost of breakfast and lunch meals for the representative baseline menus using data from SNDA-III related to the percentage of each item that was selected by the students;

4. Revised a subset of the representative baseline menus[2] according to the recommended standards for menu planning (see Chapter 7, Table 7-3) to produce *modified baseline menus*;

5. Estimated the cost of the food in breakfast and lunch meals for the modified baseline menus using estimated values for the percentage of each item that would be selected by the students; and

6. Compared the cost of the food in the set of six 5-day modified baseline menus to the subset of six 5-day representative baseline menus to assess likely effects of the proposed changes on food costs for reimbursable meals. The subset included the traditional food-based menus only.

It is important to note that the representative baseline menus were selected to be "representative;" that is, neither better nor worse than existed at the time of the survey (school year 2004–2005). Although the process used to select the representative baseline menus involved selecting from a relatively large set of candidate menus, the variability of the menu items across schools meant that some of the menus selected for the representative baseline may have had costs that were higher or lower than the average. The committee modified the representative menus by changing some food items and amounts, but only to the extent needed to meet the recommended standards for menu planning. Thus, many of the foods (and food costs) remained the same. The availability of national-level cost data from the same period allowed the committee to take advantage of relatively recent information in assessing the cost implications of modifications that reflect the recommended changes.

Matching to Cost Data

The SNDA-III study has extensive information on the meals offered by school food authorities (SFAs) and on the foods actually served (selected by the students)—including the amounts of food, nutrients in the foods, and food descriptions. However, SNDA-III has no information on costs

---

[2]The subset comprised six sets of menus (breakfast and lunch for three age-grade levels, each of which covered 5 school days) that had been planned using the existing traditional food-based method of menu planning.

or prices of the component foods. Data on the costs of specific food items from the SLBCS-II were recently released for an extensive set of food items used by SFAs (USDA/FNS, 2008g). Food items were matched at the level of food item code through a software application that was specially developed for the committee work (see Appendix K). Because the matching between the SNDA-III and SLBCS-II food items was not complete, it was necessary to develop additional food price information for food items included in the representative baseline menus and the modified baseline menus. When needed, estimates of the cost of food were imputed using similar products, component products (e.g., adding ingredients such as lettuce to a cheese sandwich), or (if needed in a very limited number of cases) 2005–2006 records from actual food service units. The 2005–2006 school year was considered the base period for analysis.

Estimating the Food Costs of Menus

For the representative baseline menus, the committee used information on each food item included, serving size (converted to grams), and cost (per 100 g) to estimate the cost per food item. The SNDA-III data on the representative baseline menus also include the number of servings of each food item and the number of reimbursable meals served for each of the menu days. To account for the percentage of the food items selected by students, a percent *take-up* was estimated for each food item based on the number of servings as a share of total reimbursable meals. The cost of each of the representative baseline meals *as offered* by the school was estimated using "offer" weights in the SNDA-III data.[3] The food cost of the reimbursed meal was estimated using the estimated percent take-up values for each food item to weight the cost aggregated over all the food items served.

For the modified baseline menus, the assignment of offered weights used the method employed in the SNDA-III study, which was based on a simple average of each of the required meal components. However, because student selection (take-up) rates cannot be known in advance of offering a meal, the method for the assignment of the rates used to estimate the reimbursed food costs required the use of assumptions. To consider the uncertainties about the assignment of take-up rates for the modified baseline menus, the committee conducted two analyses. The specific values used and the rationale for their use in the first analysis may be found in Tables L-1 through L-6 in Appendix L. Quality control measures were in place to ensure accurate data entry.

[3]The SNDA-III offer weights were designed to produce a simple average of nutrient content (or, in this case, costs), assuming that meals included an average serving from each of the required meal components (milk, vegetable/fruit, meat, and grain), based on existing Meal Requirements.

For the first analysis of the reimbursed food costs, the committee assigned take-up rates that reflected *offer versus serve* (OVS) opportunities and expected student preferences (based on current patterns) as described below. In brief, the first analysis generated a set of cost estimates that assumed a moderate increase in student's selection of fruits and vegetables. Table 8-3 indicates the approximate amount of change in the assigned take-up rates that were used in the first analysis, by food group.

The take-up rates that the committee assigned for the first analysis were based on evidence from SNDA-III and on expert judgment from current school meal practitioners. However, the committee recognized that take-up rates for fruits and vegetables could increase substantially with very effective implementation strategies. To address this possibility, the committee's second analysis assigned take-up rates for fruits and vegetables that were substantially higher than those shown in Table 8-3. The rates that were used in the second analysis appear in Table L-7 in Appendix L.

For both the representative and the modified baseline menus, the cost of the breakfast meal and lunch meal was estimated both by school level (elementary, middle, and high school) and aggregated across all school levels. The total aggregates across the school levels include *total unweighted averages* (estimated with equal contributions from the three school levels) and *total weighted averages* (with the meal cost values weighted by the

TABLE 8-3 Analysis I. Change in Assigned Take-up Rates[a] Relative to Rates in Data from the Third School Nutrition Dietary Assessment Study (SNDA-III), by Food Group

Food Group	Assigned Take-up Rates Compared with SNDA-III Data
Fluid milk	No change
Meat/meat alternates	No change
Grains	No change
Fruits	50% increase at breakfast, no change at elementary or middle school lunch,[a] 50% increase at high school lunch over rates observed in schools that allowed 2 fruit servings[b]
Vegetables	Comparable to rates for schools that allowed students to take 2 vegetables (an average of 1.1 to 1.3 servings of vegetables per child)[c]

[a]Actual take-up rates used vary with age-grade group and meal, but the changes are comparable across the age-grade groups. Specific values used may be found in Tables L-1 through L-6 in Appendix L.

[b]Fruits are popular; average take-up rate used for both was 80 percent.

[c]Further increases in total take-up rates for vegetables were not assumed because the most popular vegetables (French fries, corn) are offered less often under the recommended standards for menu planning, and take-up rates for most other vegetables in SNDA-III were very low.

average number of meals served in the schools at each level, based on the distribution of meals in the SNDA-III study).

ESTIMATED CHANGES IN FOOD COSTS FOR MODIFIED MENUS

The estimated food costs of the complete set of representative baseline menus, the subset of food-based representative baseline menus, and the modified food-based representative baseline menus are shown in Table 8-4, along with the estimated percentage change from baseline.

Cost of Food in Representative Baseline Menus

Using elementary school lunch and the food- and nutrient-based representative baseline menus as an example, the food cost *as offered* by the school was $1.17 per meal, and as reimbursed (selected by the student) was $1.06 per meal. Over all age-grade levels, the average (weighted) lunch food costs *as offered* were higher ($1.26 per meal); and the average (weighted) lunch food costs *as selected* were lower ($0.98 per meal) when compared with the elementary school. For comparison, the average lunch food cost for meals served in the SLBCS-II national survey for the same period was $1.09 per meal when the unit of analysis was the SFA, and $0.98 when the unit of analysis was the reimbursable meal. Of note, the SFA-based analysis gives more weight to smaller school units.

The estimated average baseline cost of the breakfast meal (the food- and nutrient-based baseline menus) was $0.60 per meal as reimbursed. This cost compares to the reference food cost of $0.73 per meal when the unit of analysis is the SFA and $0.65 per meal when the unit of analysis is the reimbursable meal. The average food costs for the representative baseline menu and reference SLBCS-II study confirm that the baseline menus are representative in food costs. The estimated food cost for the baseline breakfast meal is slightly lower than the reference value.

Food Costs of Modified Baseline Menus Compared with Representative Baseline Menus

The modified baseline food costs were compared with the appropriate baseline food costs *as offered* and as reimbursed. To evaluate the effect of the recommended Meal Requirements, the cost of the modified baseline menus was compared to the cost of the food-based representative baseline menu. The representative baseline menus were representative of both the types and amounts of food items offered by the SFAs.

TABLE 8-4 Average Food Cost of Reimbursable Meals, as Reimbursed and Offered (2005–2006 dollar values)

		Baseline Menus (food- and nutrient-based menus)[a]* n = 60		Baseline Menus (food-based only)[a]* n = 30		Modified Baseline Menus[b] n = 30		Percent of Baseline (food-based only)	
		Cost of Meal ($)						Cost (%)	
Meal	Level	Offered	Reimbursed[c]	Offered	Reimbursed[c]	Offered	Reimbursed[c]	Offered	Reimbursed[c,d,e]
Breakfast	Elementary	0.67	0.64	0.74	0.72	0.81	0.69	108.3	95.6
	Middle	0.59	0.58	0.53	0.50	0.81	0.65	151.5	130.9
	High	0.70	0.59	0.54	0.56	1.03	0.82	189.0	146.2
	Total (unweighted)[f]	0.65	0.60	0.61	0.59	0.88	0.72	145.0	121.3
	Total (weighted)[g]	0.66	0.60	0.62	0.61	0.87	0.72	140.5	118.2
	Reference, Unit of Analysis SFA[h]**		0.73						
	Reference, Unit of Analysis is Reimbursable Meal[h]**		0.65						
Lunch	Elementary	1.17	1.06	0.94	0.83	1.00	0.82	107.0	98.1
	Middle	1.32	0.87	1.36	0.89	1.05	0.87	77.6	97.3
	High	1.28	1.01	1.26	1.01	1.37	1.18	108.5	116.8
	Total (unweighted)[f]	1.26	0.98	1.19	0.91	1.14	0.96	96.4	104.8
	Total (weighted)[g]	1.26	0.98	1.18	0.91	1.13	0.94	95.4	104.0
	Reference, Unit of Analysis SFA[h]**		1.09						
	Reference, Unit of Analysis is Reimbursable Meal[h]**		0.98						

NOTE: See Appendix K for the number of meals used for weights.

[a]Representative baseline menus selected from SNDA-III data, as described in Appendix L.

[b]Revised versions of the food-based representative baseline menus, modified to be consistent with the recommended standards for menu planning.

[c]The term "reimbursed" refers to meals *as selected* by the students (meals *as served*).

[d]If the number of food items served for each food is restricted to 100 percent of the number of meals offered, the food costs for breakfast increases to 120.4 percent of the baseline cost and the cost for lunch increases to 104.4 percent of the baseline cost for food.

[e]If the elementary school is restricted to no OVS, the cost of the elementary breakfast *as selected* increases to 112.5 percent of the baseline cost; the cost of elementary lunch *as selected* increases to 119.4 percent. Restricting the elementary meals to no-OVS leads to an overall (weighted) cost increase of 126.3 percent for breakfast and 110.8 percent for lunch.

[f]The estimated cost of elementary modified baseline menus differs between offered and reimbursed, but after rounding to two-digits, they are equal. The more limited selections at the elementary school level result in similar costs for the modified baseline menus.

[g]Mean food costs for meals across grade levels weighted by average meals served.

[h]Reference value from SLBCS-II (USDA/FNS, 2008f).

SOURCES: *Represents costs for meals planned using only the food-based menu planning approach from SNDA-III (USDA/FNS, 2007a); cost of food items from USDA/FNS, 2008g. SLBCS-II costs were supplemented by those for similar foods and from food service records. Reference values for food costs, SLBCS-II Tables Exhibit D.8, D.9, D.11, D.12 (USDA/FNS, 2008f). **Represents reported costs of producing a reimbursable meal from the School Lunch and Breakfast Cost Study (USDA/FNS, 2008f).

Results of Analysis One

Using the first set of assumptions about take-up rates, comparison of the food costs for the modified baseline menu with those of the representative baseline menu for lunch and breakfast shows that, in general, the food costs increased significantly. The increase was most marked for breakfast: an average of 40 percent for the offered breakfast meal and 18 percent for the meal *as selected* (as reimbursed). One caveat, as noted previously, is that the food costs of the representative baseline breakfast menus were slightly lower (about $0.05 per meal) than the reference value taken from the SLBCS-II study. However, even accounting for this small difference (7 to 8 percent of the cost), the food cost of the modified breakfast meal is estimated to be higher.

- The food cost of the modified elementary breakfast is quite comparable to the baseline (modified is higher *as offered*, but not *as selected*). The increase in fruits is offset by decreases in the cost of other menu items. When the elementary students have no OVS option,[4] the food cost of the breakfast would be 12 percent higher than the representative baseline level. Requiring elementary students to take more fruit servings would increase breakfast costs.
- Food costs for the middle and high school meals are higher in the modified breakfast meals. The main reason for the increase in food costs at breakfast is the addition of a fruit serving and grain product servings (including whole grain-rich foods) for all levels, and of meat or meat alternates to meet the recommended standard for menu planning.
- For lunch, there is some variability across the modified baseline food costs. Overall, the modified baseline lunch menus were slightly lower in food cost *as offered* (95 percent of the baseline) and slightly higher in costs *as selected* (104 percent of the baseline). Higher student selection of foods and increased costs for foods on the modified menu increased costs for meals *as selected*, especially for the high school menus.
- The food cost for the high school lunch meal increased more than the cost of the elementary and middle school meals. The addition of more fruit and vegetables, more varied vegetables, and whole grain-rich foods (especially at the high school level) increased costs. The increase in costs at the high school level came despite offering starchy vegetables less often and a smaller amount of meat and meat alternates.

The evaluation of the cost of food in the modified baseline menus indicates that offering menus consistent with the recommended standards for

[4]In the case of OVS, the student is required to select the full amount of food.

menu planning is likely to increase the cost of the school meals, especially for breakfast. For the menus used in the analysis, the food costs for breakfast (*as selected*) increased up to 18 percent; for lunch (*as selected*), they increased by about 4 percent.

Results of Analysis Two

In the second analysis, take-up rates were assigned that assumed that students selected more fruits and vegetables. The increase in foods selected comes at a higher cost. There is no change between the baseline menus and modified baseline costs *as offered* because the menus themselves for this comparison do not change, only the student selection. When students select more fruits at breakfast, the food cost of the meal is significantly higher than the baseline values. With the assumption of increased fruits selected at breakfast, the elementary school breakfast food costs increase by 3 percentage points over the costs estimated in analysis one. For the middle school menus, the costs are 37 percent higher than the baseline (6 percentage points higher than for the modified baseline cost that assumed lower take-up rates for fruits and vegetables). For the high school breakfasts, the overall increase is almost 52 percent higher than the baseline (and 6 percentage points higher than for the modified baseline cost from analysis one). Overall, the breakfast food costs increase almost 5 percentage points over the modified baseline food costs for breakfast estimated in analysis one.

For lunch, the changes are similar when the results of analysis two are compared with those from analysis one. The increased selection of fruits and vegetables increases the food costs of the middle school lunch by 3 percentage points and for high school by about 6 percentage points. The elementary lunch food costs increase by 5 percentage points. Overall, the lunch costs increase 5 percentage points over the cost increases of the modified baseline food costs that assumed lower take-up rates for fruits and vegetables.

Summary of Changes in Estimated Food Costs of Modified Menus

Table 8-5 summarizes the percentage increases in the reimbursed food costs of school meals under the two sets of assumptions for student take-up rates for the selected menus. Some of the estimated changes may be smaller than anticipated because the estimates are influenced by several factors, a selection of which is presented in Box 8-1.

TABLE 8-5 Estimated Increases in Reimbursed Food Costs for Modified Menus

Analysis	Assumptions about Student Take-up Rates	Breakfast	Lunch
		% increase in food costs	
1	Moderate increase in fruit and vegetable selection	18	4
2	More optimistic increase in fruit and vegetable selection	23	9

Limitations of Cost Comparison Method

It is important to note that although the take-up rates that were assigned by the committee for use in analysis one were based on current (baseline) evidence as well as expert judgment from current school meal practitioners, there is some uncertainty about the expected values, given change under the full set of recommendations. In addition, the food items included in the representative baseline menus were those actually offered to students in the survey year. There was no restriction that the number of food items be only those required. Any additional offering would have the effect of increasing the foods, nutrients, and costs of the representative baseline menus. Also, the estimated costs are based on food item costs

BOX 8-1
Reasons for Change in Estimated Food Costs of School Meals Assuming the Adoption of the Recommended Meal Requirements

- Addition of fruits and vegetables, and additional meat or meat alternate[a]
  - Fruit serving (about $0.14–0.15 per serving)
  - Vegetable serving (about $0.07–0.09 per serving)
  - Meat or meat alternates (about $0.30–0.33 per serving, 2 oz)
- Substitution of foods
  - Whole grain-rich item in place of refined item (increase of 3–20 percent)
  - Foods with lower proportion of saturated fat (variable effects on the cost of the item)
- Deletion of selected foods, such as dessert items (variable cost per serving)
- Student selection of foods (change in student selection may increase or decrease food costs of the meals served)

[a]Representative costs based on 2005–2006 prices.

as reported from survey data from SFAs for the school year 2005–2006. Food prices have changed since that time (see the section "Changes in Food Prices" later in this chapter). These price changes certainly affect the level of costs reported above. Importantly, changes in the relative importance of food items that occur through the menu modifications also affect the estimated changes in food costs and hence the committee's estimates of the percentage changes. The effect of changes in food prices is discussed in the next section.

OTHER FACTORS AFFECTING MEAL COSTS

Many factors affect the price of school meals. Some directly affect the cost of food. Others relate to the food service operation. Several of these factors are discussed briefly below.

Other Factors Affecting the Cost of Food in School Meals

Food purchase practices have a major impact on the cost of food. The Phase I report (IOM, 2008) provides brief summaries of relevant findings from cost studies (USDA/FNS, 2008f) and a school food purchasing study (USDA/FNS, 1998b), along with the websites that can be accessed to obtain further information. At a minimum, procurement and purchasing regulations must conform to federal regulations found at 7 CFR 3016.36, but they are determined at the state level, and they vary considerably from state to state.

The School Cost Environment

School Food Authorities' (SFAs') food costs vary widely because of many factors, including

- Methods the state uses to manage U.S. Department of Agriculture (USDA)[5] foods (and also the amount a school district receives in USDA food values, which depends on participation the year prior);
- Purchasing rules of the state or district;
- Geographical differences that govern the availability of fresh produce, dairy products, and grain products;
- Location in metropolitan or rural area;
- Bid pricing and purchasing power;
- Quality of the bid specification;
- Distributor costs, district and distributor locations;

[5]USDA foods are known familiarly as commodity foods.

- Level of competition for the business among distributors;
- Student, geographical, or cultural food preferences; and
- Variety of cooking and production methods (for example, onsite versus central kitchen with satellite sites, convenience heat and serve versus cooking from basic ingredients).

School districts have the flexibility to change menus as needed depending on market prices, availability of product, and other factors. Nevertheless, the menus must meet the current Meal Requirements. When a major beef recall occurred in spring 2008, for example, SFAs quickly had to substitute chicken or turkey for beef. The substitutions resulted in some cost variations and difficulties in meeting the Meal Requirement for iron.

USDA manages the procurement of agricultural (food) commodities through the Agricultural Marketing Service (AMS) and the Kansas City Commodity Office of the Farm Service Agency. AMS purchases a variety of food products with the goal to stabilize the prices in agricultural commodity markets. Fresh and processed foods customarily purchased under these programs include fruit and vegetables, beef and pork, poultry and egg products, and fish. The Kansas City Commodity Office purchases grain products including pasta, processed cereal, flours, crackers, ready-to-eat cereal, rice products, corn products, and miscellaneous dairy products; and it facilitates food distribution and multifood warehouse contracts.

USDA Foods

As mentioned in the bulleted list above, the use of USDA foods affects the food costs for SFAs. A per-meal rate for USDA entitlement foods is established by law, namely Section 6 of the Richard B. Russell National School Lunch Act. This law established a guaranteed rate of 11 cents per meal to be adjusted annually for inflation. The rate is applied to the number of lunches served during the previous school year (USDA/FNS, 2008a). The rate published for school year 2009–2010 is 19.5 cents (USDA/FNS, 2009e). In addition, bonus products are made available to an extent that varies with the need to remove surplus products from the marketplace. The dollar value of the bonus products (about $17 million in fiscal year [FY] 2007) is much smaller than that of the entitlement foods (about $1.1 billion in FY 2007).

The use of USDA foods reduces costs for school meal programs in the following ways:

- The foods are provided at no cost (other than shipping and handling) to participating schools.

- The monetary value of the foods would be greater if bought on the open market, which increases the cost savings to the schools.

The value of some USDA foods relative to the open market varies, however (CFPA, 2008).

On average in school year 2005–2006, USDA foods accounted for 12 percent of the *total food costs* for SFAs (USDA/FNS, 2008f). For more than 60 percent of the SFAs, USDA foods accounted for at least 10 percent of total food costs. Some schools, however, do not use USDA foods at all (CFPA, 2008). When USDA foods are considered as a percentage of *total revenue*, however, the median is approximately 5 percent. This represents a substantial decrease since school year 1992–1993, when USDA foods accounted for 8 percent of total revenue (USDA/FNS, 2008f).

USDA Fresh Fruit and Vegetable Program

Additionally, the 2008 Farm Bill amended the *National School Lunch Act* to expand the USDA Fresh Fruit and Vegetable Program. Beginning in the 2008–2009 school year (United Fresh Produce Association, 2009), the program increased funding available for purchases of available fresh fruits and vegetables to all students throughout the day if more than 50 percent of their student enrollment in the NSLP comprised students eligible for free and reduced-price meals (*Food, Conservation, and Energy Act of 2008*, P.L. 100-246 [June 18, 2008]: § 4304).

Changes in Food Prices

Relative prices have changed since the 2006 school year, as shown in Table 8-6; but price changes over the period are not uniform across all foods. The data used for the estimates of costs in the previous section come from the USDA Cost Study data (USDA/FNS, 2008f). This national survey was conducted during the 2005–2006 school year. Between 2006 and 2009, on average, overall food prices rose 12.2 percent. (The yearly average over this period is just over 4 percent.) Prices for food at home rose 12.1 percent, and prices for food away from home rose 12.4 percent during the 3-year period.

Food prices reflect varying market conditions,[6] however; and, in the

[6]Agricultural programs and policies are among the factors that affect food prices, but the relative magnitude of the effects tends to be small and varies across foods. For example, farm subsidies and other agricultural policies in the United States have increased dairy and orange juice prices and decreased cereal, bread, and meat prices (Alston et al., 2006, 2008); and today they have little effect on sweetened products (Beghin and Jensen, 2008). Although changes in farm subsidies could have an effect on the relative prices of certain foods purchased

TABLE 8-6 Percentage Change in the Consumer Price Index for All Urban Consumers (May)

Item	2006–2007	2007–2008	2008–2009
All Food	3.9	5.1	2.7
Food at home	4.4	5.8	1.5
Food away from home	3.3	4.3	4.2
Bakery products	4.6	11.1	6.6
Dairy and related	3.5	11.0	3.1
Fluid milk	7.5	10.2	–5.6
Eggs	29.6	18.2	–13.6
Meat	4.7	0.53	–17.8
Fruit and vegetable (F&V)	6.7	4.4	1.8
Fresh F&V	7.7	3.3	–4.1
Processed F&V	2.9	8.4	9.9

NOTES: Adjustment for 2007–2008 School Meal Programs was 4.272 percent. This percentage change differs from the number for Food away from home reported here (4.256 percent) due to rounding.
SOURCE: U.S. Bureau of Labor Statistics, 2008.

2007–2009 period, there was substantial volatility in food prices. For example, the cost of food at home increased 5.8 percent between 2007 and 2008 but increased only 1.5 percent between 2008 and 2009 (see Table 8-6). Between May[7] 2006 and May 2008, the prices of bakery items, dairy foods, eggs, and processed fruits and vegetables rose at a faster rate than did the prices of many other food items. Between 2008 and 2009, however, several types of foods fell in price. The prices of meat and eggs fell dramatically in the 2008–2009 period. The prices of processed fruits and vegetables increased at a rate faster than other foods during the latest two-year periods. Thus, in the current food environment, school districts must make significant adjustments to accommodate dramatic changes in price. For some years, they must make adjustments for rapidly rising costs for some key foods, such as eggs and meat.

Other changes may also affect the costs that school units pay for food. For example, new foods and packaging continue to change costs. As these new food products are developed and made available in the market, the school food directors will weigh the full set of costs in selecting the food products. Changes in school procurement procedures also affect costs. In Minnesota, for example, the school districts that participate in a Joint

by school food authorities, the magnitude of the effect is likely to be small and affected by a wide range of other government programs, including research and development funding and trade policies.

[7]May is the month of adjustment for the School Meal Programs.

Powers Agreement have access to better purchasing power through the increased size of the buyer negotiating unit. This type of agreement can make purchasing more competitive for smaller districts or smaller states. Increased packaging (single serving units, for example) may increase the cost of the unit value to the school but may reduce waste and labor costs.

Labor, Administrative, and Equipment Costs

Several factors influence comparisons of the costs of the *meals* (not just the foods) that are provided under the current and recommended Meal Requirements. The major factors include changes in labor, administrative, and equipment costs.

Average Costs

Based on data from (USDA/FNS, 2008f), *reported* costs to operate the National School Lunch Program (NSLP) and the School Breakfast Program (SBP) include

- food costs, about 46 percent;
- labor costs, about 45 percent; and
- other costs (supplies, contract services, and indirect charges by school districts), about 10 percent of the total cost.

For the average SFA, the national mean reported SFA costs of producing a reimbursable breakfast and a reimbursable lunch and the mean meal cost of the SBP and NSLP meals are shown in Table 8-7. The table does not provide data on the variability of meal costs, which may be substantial

TABLE 8-7 Comparison of the *Reported* Costs of Producing a Reimbursable Meal, SBP and NSLP, by Unit of Analysis, 2005–2006 School Year

	SBP		NSLP	
Type of Cost	Mean SFA Cost	Mean Meal Cost	Mean SFA Cost	Mean Meal Cost
Reported[a]	$1.92	$1.46	$2.36	$2.28
Food	$0.73	$0.65	$1.09	$0.98
Labor	$1.02	$0.64	$1.05	$1.04
Other	$0.17	$0.17	$0.23	$0.25

NOTES: NSLP = National School Lunch Program; SBP = School Breakfast Program; SFA = School Food Authority.

[a]Reported costs may not equal the sum of the component costs because of rounding.

SOURCE: USDA/FNS, 2008f.

during a week or even within a year. It is important to note that reported costs include only those costs charged to the SFA budgets. The full cost of producing a reimbursable meal would also include costs incurred by the school district that support the SFA operations but are not charged (or reported) as costs to the SFA and, if applicable, transfers of local educational money to cover food service budget losses in excess of program fund balance (USDA/FNS, 2008f).

Using either unit of analysis (mean SFA cost or mean meal cost), the food and labor costs represented most (approximately 90 percent) of the average *reported* costs. *Full* costs, which include costs incurred but not charged to the SFA, are higher for both lunch and breakfast.

The food costs and the associated reported labor and administrative costs shown in Table 8-7 have been used to provide a benchmark for estimated school meal costs. In addition, indirect costs for labor, equipment, and other items that may not be reported add to the cost of providing school meals. These indirect costs also have been investigated (USDA/FNS, 2008f) and used to determine the *full* cost of the meals. Importantly, considerable variation has been observed across SFA by size and other factors (USDA/FNS, 2008f).

Although these costs are reported on the basis of average meal costs, ultimately, SFAs establish costs and resolve the reimbursement process at the end of a menu cycle and at the end of the school year. Hence, for planning purposes, there may be considerable variability in costs on a specific day or week.

Changes in the Distribution of Costs of Preparing Reimbursable Meals

One possible approach to offering school meals that meet the recommended standards for menu planning is to introduce more on-site food preparation. This approach requires greater managerial skill, often requires substantial one-time investment in equipment, and most often would require more skilled labor and/or training (Wagner et al., 2007). Such an approach would be consistent with USDA's new "Know Your Farmer, Know Your Food Initiative," which has the goal of assisting school administrators to purchase more locally grown foods.

An empirical analysis of data from 330 Minnesota school districts found that "healthier" meals had higher labor costs (for on-site preparation) but lower costs for processed foods (Wagner et al., 2007). The authors call for funds to be made available for labor training and kitchen upgrades. They suggest that higher federal meal reimbursement rates may be unnecessary (under the assumption that the meals do not cost more to produce because lower food costs offset higher labor costs).

Opportunities for on-site preparation also influenced the choice of foods to include in the modified menus. Successfully adhering to the recommended changes in the Meal Requirements may result in changes in indirect costs for labor, equipment, and other items that may not be reported. An overview of ways to control the cost of school meals is presented in Chapter 10.

Student Acceptance

Student acceptance of the meals and selection of the foods that are offered is an important consideration to the costs of meals and is reflected in the percent take-up of any specific food item. More generally, however, a change in the meal offered may induce more (or fewer) students to participate in the school meal program, as discussed in Chapter 9. Another possible effect might be the participation of more (or fewer) students who pay the full price of the meal. Changes in student participation in the school meal programs have not been addressed in the analysis of costs presented here.

OVERALL IMPACT OF THE RECOMMENDED MEAL REQUIREMENTS ON THE COSTS OF SCHOOL MEALS

The food cost analyses clearly indicate that the recommended changes in the Meal Requirements increase the cost of the food used in school meals. Because of the many variables involved, the committee had no practical way to estimate the impact of the recommendations on the full cost of the meals. The committee recognizes that, at current reimbursement levels, most school food authorities will be unable to absorb these increased food costs completely, even with better management. However, some might be able to do so if they have the capability to use fewer highly processed foods. Implementation of the recommended Meal Requirements likely will require some combination of higher federal meal reimbursement, a source of capital investment to cover initial costs of equipment, and additional money to train operators to prepare more food from basic ingredients.

ECONOMIC IMPACT AND IMPLICATIONS FOR COMMODITY MARKETS

The school meal programs represent a major buyer of the food supply in the United States, and changes to the programs hold the potential for significant impacts in agricultural markets. The SBP and NSLP represent half of all food costs spent on child nutrition programs (USDA/ERS, 2003).

The current requirements for food-based menu planning and the recommended changes for breakfast and for lunch are summarized in Tables 8-1 and 8-2. For the breakfast meal (Table 8-1), the recommendations provide for changes in the amounts of fruit, grain/bread products, and meat and meat alternates. Unlike the current requirements for breakfast, the recommendations determine that half of the grain/bread products should be whole grain rich (see Box 7-1 in Chapter 7 for the whole grain-rich food criterion). For the lunch meal (Table 8-2), the recommended menus include an aggregate increase in the amount of fruits and vegetables, with increased variety for vegetables, and an increase in the amount of grain products. Grain products include half whole grain-rich products.

The changes presented in Tables 8-1 and 8-2 indicate that the school meal programs would increase their use of some foods, decrease the use of other foods, and have little change in others. In some cases, the composition of the food would need to change (such as the use of low-fat or fat-free milk in place of higher fat milks) in order to meet *Dietary Guidelines*.

Table 8-8 provides values for an upper bound of assumed changes in the amounts of foods recommended by food type, for a 5-day school week, for the purpose of assessing market effects. These changes are based on the difference between the amounts of foods offered under the new recommendations and the amounts in the current requirements. Changes in amounts were estimated by assuming the current requirements to be represented in the average of menu plans (traditional food-based menus, nutrient-based and enhanced food-based) that is recorded by the SNDA-III data. For each food type, the change in the amount offered was calculated as the difference between the recommended levels and the current (average) levels. Additional assumptions were used to distribute the food item over the more disaggregated types of food in the recommended menus.

The amounts in the table represent an upper bound for weekly change because they are based on the standards for menu planning. In the large majority of schools that have OVS, the amount of each food that is actually offered is based on the operator's knowledge of the foods the students have selected in the past. (Under OVS, students are permitted to decline a specified number of food items—many do so, and this would be the case under the recommended menus as well. For more information on OVS, see Chapters 5 and 7, including Table 7-4.) Also, some schools had already taken steps to add fruits, a variety of vegetables, and whole grain-rich foods to their menus in 2004–2005. The changes in menus required to meet the recommendations would be smaller for these schools than for the average SFA.

For the breakfast meal, the greatest change in foods is the increase in fruit, which doubles from the current requirement. If all students were to take only one fruit or fruit juice, the amount of fruit provided would still increase significantly from current practice. Grains increase significantly over current levels, with a shift to whole grains. For the lunch meal, the

TABLE 8-8 Upper Bound of Assumed Changes in Amounts of Foods Recommended by Food Type, for a 5-Day School Week, for the Purpose of Assessing Market Effects[a]

Food Group	Changes to Amounts Recommended		
	K–Grade 5	Grades 6–8	Grades 9–12
	Breakfast		
Fruit (cups)[b]	+2.5	+2.5	+2.5
Vegetables (cups)	0	0	0
Grain/Bread (oz eq)[c]	+3.5	+3.5	+4
Refined Grain	0	0	
Whole Grain	+3.5	+3.5	
Meat/Meat Alternates (oz eq)[d]	+0–5	+0–5	+0–10
Milk (cups)[e]	nc	nc	nc
	Lunch		
Fruit (cups)	+1–2	+1–2	+3–4
Vegetables (cups)[f,g,h]	+1–2	+1–2	+2–3
Dark Green	(+)	(+)	(+)
Orange	(+)	(+)	(+)
Legumes	(+)	(+)	(+)
Starchy	(–)	(–)	(–)
Other	(+)	(+)	(+)
Grain/Bread (oz eq)	nc	nc	nc
Refined Grain	(–)	(–)	(–)
Whole Grain	(+)	(+)	(+)
Meat/Meat Alternates (oz eq)[i,j]	+1–2	nc	–1–2
Milk (cups)	nc	nc	nc

NOTES: Weighted estimates of changes assume 48 percent of schools are traditional (food-based) planning; 52 percent other (nutrient based or enhanced). K = kindergarten; nc = no change; oz eq = ounce equivalent.

[a]The assumed changes were used to guide qualitative assessment of market effects.

[b]These are recommended amounts offered for breakfast. Under Preferred Option 1 (Table 7-4), student may decline one item, but must take one fruit or juice.

[c]Assume, under current requirements, 12.5 percent of grains are whole grain or whole grain-rich foods for food-based planning, and 25 percent are whole grain or whole grain-rich for nutrient based and enhanced. This implies that, on average, 18.75 percent of the required grain items are whole grain or whole grain-rich (for each 5 ounces, approximately 1 ounce meets the whole grain target).

[d]Assume 20 percent of increase is meat alternates (cheese, yogurt).

[e]Although there is no change in the recommended amount of milk, the composition changes with milk choices limited to fat-free (plain or flavored) and plain low-fat (1 percent or less). Some reduction in milk may occur.

[f]These are recommended amounts offered for lunch. Under Preferred Option 1 (Table 7-4), the student may decline two items but must take one fruit or vegetable.

[g]Assume the increase in fruits and vegetables is through 60 percent increase in fruits, 40 percent increase in vegetables.

[h]Increase in vegetables to meet the requirement of increased variety in vegetables at the same time as a reduction of starchy vegetables.

[i]Assume 20 percent of increase for K–5 is meat alternates (beans, cheese, yogurt).

[j]Assume 20 percent of decrease for high school is meat alternates (beans, cheese, yogurt).

largest change is the increased offering of fruits and vegetables, an increase of nearly four half-cup servings a week. Although it is not known what choices students will make if allowed to decline two foods but required to select at least one fruit or vegetable, SNDA-III data suggest that they will be more likely to select fruit. The increase in vegetables involves an increase in the variety of vegetables and a reduction of popular starchy vegetables such as white potatoes and corn.

The increase in foods offered through the program can have important effects on some markets. Based on a review of the literature, Hanson (USDA/ERS, 2003) estimates that the NSLP generates an additional 45 percent of food consumption and that the SBP generates an additional 73 percent of food consumption—that is, the value of added food consumption generated by a program after netting food that would have been consumed anyway (USDA/ERS, 2003). For the school meal programs, about half of those additional food expenditures come directly from farm production (cash receipts). The amount and percentage of change noted in Table 8-8 suggest that the greatest changes will be for increased fruits and vegetables. Buzby and colleagues (USDA/ERS, 2006) review similar implications for U.S. agricultural markets that would arise from the adoption of *Dietary Guidelines* in current consumption patterns.

For fruits and vegetables, the effects are likely to vary by production region, with fruit production more highly concentrated in a few states (e.g., California, Florida, Washington) and vegetable production more widely dispersed. The consumption of fruits and vegetables has been increasing over several decades. Much of the national demand for fruit has been supplied by increased imports. The comparative advantage of increased domestic production of fruit, especially in the variety preferred by school age children, is limited by land and water availability as well as climate (USDA/ERS, 2006). Hence, increased demand for fruit is likely to face continuing higher prices. Increased vegetable and legume production faces fewer limitations on acreage and, hence, on expanding domestic supplies.

The major impact on grain markets is the shift from refined grain products to whole grain-rich products. Although the range of options available for whole grains includes oats, brown rice, and other grains, most of the change is likely to come with the development and use of additional wheat products made with whole grain. Whole grain products use somewhat less grain ingredient than do refined grain product (less diverted through milling) (USDA/ERS, 2006), but the slight increase in grain product demand would likely offset the small losses from changes in milling. Of greater concern is the relative lack of available whole grain-rich processed products on the market and acceptable in the school meals program. Hence some cost increases would be expected for the less available processed whole grain-rich products in the market. Several new whole grain products are being introduced through the USDA foods program; over time, the availability of whole grain-rich products is expected to expand.

Overall (across breakfast and lunch) relatively smaller changes in meat and dairy products were required by the recommended changes, which would suggest a more limited market impact on these sectors. However, the effort to offer students one meat or meat alternate daily at breakfast would imply some increases, especially for the meat or meat alternates. The school meal programs purchase large amounts of these products (USDA/FNS, 1998b). Although no change is expected in the amount of milk offered, the stricter limitations on the type of milk (to low-fat and fat-free varieties) and on saturated fat (shift to reduced-fat cheeses, for example) may put some upward pressure on lower fat milk varieties. However, demand for butterfat and cheese has remained relatively strong. As evidenced by the rapid rise in the cost of dairy products during the 2007–2008 period, the SFAs are vulnerable to dairy product price increases.

One of the challenges to estimating the market effect of the school meal programs is determining whether the school meal consumption *supplements* the children's consumption of certain foods (that is, increases their intake of those foods during the day) or *substitutes* for foods that may have been consumed at other times during the day. With supplementation, the market effects described above would be most strongly experienced. With substitution, there would be few market effects (this would occur, for example, if students who eat more fruit from school meals would eat less fruit at home).

SUMMARY

To examine the expected change in food costs of offering menus consistent with the recommended standards for menu planning, the committee compared the estimated cost of modified baseline menus with those of representative baseline menus, using likely take-up rates for the modified menus. As expected because of increases in fruits, vegetables, and whole grain-rich foods, implementation of the recommendations is likely to increase the cost of the school meals, especially for breakfast. For the selected menus, the food costs for breakfast (*as selected* by the student) increased up to 18 percent and for lunch (*as selected*) increased by 4 percent in the first analysis, which assumed moderate increases in students' selection.

For the changes recommended, market effects are expected to be the greatest for fruits, both because of higher expected supplementation in the breakfast program and because of limited domestic production. Other increased demand in the more limited markets for whole grain products, lower fat options for processed meats and entrées, and lower sodium options will present challenges to SFAs.

9

Projected Impact of the Recommended Nutrient Targets and Meal Requirements

The committee considered its four criteria (see Box 2-2 in Chapter 2) in evaluating the projected impact of its recommendations for the School Breakfast Program and the National School Lunch Program (NSLP). The recommendations considered here are those for the revision of the current Nutrition Standards (to Nutrient Targets) and of the Meal Requirements (the standards for menu planning and the standards for meals *as selected* by the student). The purpose of this evaluation is to critically examine the committee's recommendations with respect to likely benefits and negative consequences. Thus, the results may be interpreted as a sensitivity analysis. The committee notes, however, that evidence on which to base predictions of many of the effects is severely limited.

CRITERION 1: ALIGNMENT WITH *DIETARY GUIDELINES FOR AMERICANS* AND THE DIETARY REFERENCE INTAKES

The committee considered the alignment of the Meal Requirements with dietary guidance solely on the basis of the meals *as offered*. The committee recognizes that it is the food that is consumed that affects nutritional status, and it developed the standards for menu planning with student acceptability in mind. Because effective implementation of the standards will be crucial to improving student's actual consumption, Chapter 10 addresses that topic.

Methods of Evaluating Alignment with Dietary Guidance

The committee examined how well the recommended standards for menu planning and the menus themselves aligned with *Dietary Guidelines* and the Dietary Reference Intakes (DRIs). To examine the change in alignment of the standards with food-specific *Dietary Guidelines*, the committee compared the recommended meal patterns with those specified in the current Meal Requirements (see Tables 8-1 and 8-2 in Chapter 8), reviewed the food items in the modified baseline and sample menus to verify their correspondence with the *Dietary Guidelines*, and also compared the recommended standards with recommendations for children in the *Dietary Guidelines* (see Appendix P).

Examination of the alignment with the DRIs included analysis of the breakfast and lunch menus for each age-grade group, using the School Meals Menu Analysis program (Appendix K), to determine their consistency with the recommended Nutrient Targets. (The Nutrient Targets were largely based on the DRIs.) The analysis covered 6 sets of modified baseline menus (5 menus for each meal and age-grade group) and 24 sets of sample menus (20 menus for each meal and age-grade group. The committee had written these menus using the new standards for menu planning.

The committee recognizes a number of limitations of the nutrient analyses of the sample menus, as identified below, and emphasizes that operators should not be asked to conduct comparable analyses.

- The list of foods in the School Meals Menu Analysis program was limited in that it did not include a number of products with improved fat profiles that became available after the third School Nutrition Dietary Assessment study (SNDA-III).
- When exact matches for the newer foods were not found, other foods were selected to provide as close a match as possible.
- Commercial products listed in the database may not offer the same nutrient content of similar items specifically created for Child Nutrition (CN) programs, such as CN-labeled products.
- Similar items from different manufacturers may differ slightly in nutrient content; for example, sodium content may vary in different brands of chicken patties.
- Industry partners frequently adjust ingredients and recipes to meet customer requests.

Nonetheless, the committee considers the analysis adequate to show approximately how well the standards for meal planning lead to menus that come close to the Nutrient Targets. Using existing USDA-approved software, operators will be able to obtain very good estimates of the calorie, saturated fat, and sodium content of their menus; but the software would not provide information on all the nutrients. The software the committee used is not suitable for use by school food service operators. This analysis was done only to show the correspondence of the standards for meal planning with the Nutrient Targets.

The committee also considered data on nutrient contents for meals *as offered* by the school, using averages from SNDA-III (USDA/FNS, 2007a) and from the representative baseline menus described in Chapter 6. (These averages were from menus that had been planned under the existing Meal Requirements.)

Findings Regarding Alignment with Dietary Guidance

Alignment with Dietary Guidelines for Americans

The use of the recommended Meal Requirements clearly improves alignment with the *Dietary Guidelines*. Tables 8-1 and 8-2 in Chapter 8, which compare current food-based menu standards with the committee's recommendations, shows that the amounts of fruits, total vegetables, and whole grain-rich foods are substantially higher in the new meal patterns. In addition, milk products are the types encouraged in the *Dietary Guidelines*. Appendix P shows how the recommended Meal Requirements respond to each of the relevant recommendations in the *Dietary Guidelines*. The committee's review of the modified baseline menus and sample menus (which gave special attention to the inclusion of a variety of fruits and vegetables, whole grain-rich products, and fat-free or low-fat milk products) found that these menus are consistent with the food-specific *Dietary Guidelines*. The committee's recommendation that students be required to select at least one fruit at breakfast and at least one fruit or vegetable at lunch (see Table 7-4 in Chapter 7) may contribute to an increase in the consumption of foods from these important food groups. Notably, the meals contain relatively high amounts of most nutrients for the calories, as explained in the section "Effects of Nutrient Intake Contributions from School Meals on Total Daily Nutrient Intakes."

For the menus written by the committee, analysis shows that the saturated fat content as a percentage of calories (shown in Tables 9-1 through 9-3) is less than the maximum amount recommended in the *Dietary Guidelines*. Moreover, options that are high in saturated fat are minimized, meaning that students would be unable to choose higher fat forms of milk and seldom would have an option for an entrée that is high in saturated fat. In its review of data from SNDA-III (USDA/FNS, 2007a), the committee had observed that the percentage of schools *serving* meals (*as selected* by students) that met the standard for saturated fat (less than 10 percent of

TABLE 9-1 Comparison of Nutrient Values for Menus from SNDA-III Dietary Data and from Menus Planned by the Committee with Recommended Nutrient Targets for the National School Breakfast and Lunch Programs, Elementary School (children ages 5–10 years)

	Breakfast				
	Content Based on *As Offered* Menu Plans				
Nutrient (unit)	SNDA-III Mean[a*]	Rep. Baseline Menu[b*]	Modified Baseline Menu[c]	Sample Menus[d]	Nutrient Targets[e]
Calories (kcal)	463	493	452	458	350–500
Saturated Fat (g)	4	5.4	3.4	3.1	
Saturated Fat (% of kcal)	8.6	9.9	6.7	6.0	< 10
Protein (g)	15	18	21	18	10
Vitamin A (μg RAE)	242	272	268	251	129
Vitamin C (mg)	30	25	46	41	16
Vitamin E (mg αT)	0.9	0.9	*1.1*	*1.1*	2.0
Thiamin (mg)	0.5	0.44	0.41	0.39	0.25
Riboflavin (mg)	0.8	0.87	0.84	0.87	0.31
Niacin (mg)	5.0	4.2	4.5	3.8	3.2
Vitamin B_6 (mg)	0.5	0.40	0.56	0.59	0.27
Folate (μg DFE)	173	166	161	170	91
Vitamin B_{12} (μg)	1.9	1.7	2.1	2.4	0.8
Iron (mg)	4.3	4.5	4.5	3.6	2.3
Magnesium (mg)	63	69	98	87	49
Zinc (mg)	3.0	3.1	3.9	3.5	2.0
Calcium (mg)	409	464	560	529	223
Phosphorus (mg)	397	493	523	496	242
Potassium (mg)	711	757	973	957	909
Sodium (mg)	575	699	**643**	**478**	≤ 430
Linoleic Acid (g)	2.0	1.7	*1.4*	*1.6*	2.2
α-Linolenic Acid (g)	0.2	0.20	*0.16*	*0.17*	0.21
Fiber (g)	3	4	6	*4*	6

NOTES: αT = α-tocopherol; DFE = dietary folate equivalent; g = gram; mg = milligram; RAE = retinol activity equivalent; SNDA-III = third School Nutrition Dietary Assessment study; μg = microgram. Italic font indicates values that do not meet the Nutrient Targets. Bold font indicates values that exceed the maximum Nutrient Target.

[a]The menus reported in SNDA-III had been developed using the existing Nutrition Standards (covering only eight nutrients), the nutrient values of which are lower than those of the recommended Nutrient Targets. 109 schools provided the menus for breakfast, 126 for lunch.

[b]Representative baseline menus were chosen from menus available in SNDA-III, using the process described in the section "Testing of Revisions of Standards for Menu Planning" in Chapter 5, but the nutrient values of those menus were calculated by the committee. $N = 5$ menus.

Lunch				
Content Based on *As Offered* Menu Plans				
SNDA-III Mean[a]*	Rep. Baseline Menu[b]*	Modified Baseline Menu[c]	Sample Menus[d]	Nutrient Targets[f]
741	694	635	*569*	550–650
9	7.3	6.1	6.0	
10.9	9.5	8.6	*9.5*	< 10
30	28	27	27	15
294	248	439	394	192
32	24	51	38	24
2.5	2.3	3.0	*2.5*	3.0
0.5	0.51	0.41	0.40	0.37
0.9	0.95	0.81	0.80	0.46
7.0	6.2	5.3	5.3	4.7
0.5	0.55	0.62	0.52	0.40
160	137	*130*	*129*	136
1.9	1.8	2.0	2.0	1.2
4.5	4.4	4.1	3.6	3.4
102	95	120	103	72
3.8	3.7	3.8	3.7	2.9
531	520	498	486	332
571	542	592	*559*	361
1,124	1,179	*1,265*	*1,166*	1,353
1,377	1,409	**1,564**	**1,491**	≤ 640
6.0	4.2	6.4	4.1	3.3
0.7	0.46	0.58	0.37	0.31
7	6	10	7	9

[c]The committee developed the modified baseline menus by revising the representative baseline menus to meet the recommended standards for menu planning, while keeping the adjustments to a minimum. $N = 5$ menus.

[d]The committee developed the sample menus to meet the recommended standards for menu planning and to illustrate a number of different types of menus. $N = 20$ breakfast menus and 20 lunch menus for each age-grade group.

[e]Targets based on 21.5 percent of the daily School Meal-Target Median Intake (School Meal-TMI) for age-grade group.

[f]Targets based on 32 percent of the daily School Meal-TMI for the age-grade group.

SOURCE: *USDA/FNS, 2007a.

TABLE 9-2 Comparison of Nutrient Values for Menus from SNDA-III Dietary Data and from Menus Planned by the Committee with Recommended Nutrient Targets for the National School Breakfast and Lunch Programs, Middle School (children ages 11–13 years)

	Breakfast				
	Content Based on *As Offered* Menu Plans				
Nutrient (unit)	SNDA-III Mean[a]*	Rep. Baseline Menu[b]*	Modified Baseline Menu[c]	Sample Menus[d]	Nutrient Targets[e]
Calories (kcal)	501	450	510	532	400–550
Saturated Fat (g)	5	4.1	3.3	3.6	
Saturated Fat (% of kcal)	9.2	8.1	5.8	6.0	< 10
Protein (g)	16	15	*20*	*20*	22
Vitamin A (μg RAE)	257	227	251	284	162
Vitamin C (mg)	32	33	67	43	20
Vitamin E (mg αT)	1	0.85	*1.0*	*1.5*	2.7
Thiamin (mg)	0.5	0.41	0.45	0.52	0.32
Riboflavin (mg)	0.9	0.79	0.88	1.00	0.41
Niacin (mg)	5.0	3.9	4.7	5.8	4.0
Vitamin B_6 (mg)	0.5	0.43	0.50	0.78	0.36
Folate (μg DFE)	191	186	185	248	114
Vitamin B_{12} (μg)	2.0	2.1	2.1	2.9	0.9
Iron (mg)	4.6	3.6	4.6	5.1	3.5
Magnesium (mg)	64	64	83	105	66
Zinc (mg)	3.2	3.0	3.7	4.8	2.5
Calcium (mg)	432	384	468	580	296
Phosphorus (mg)	416	402	493	572	362
Potassium (mg)	730	678	*916*	1,047	1,023
Sodium (mg)	629	591	**685**	**605**	≤ 470
Linoleic Acid (g)	3.0	2.1	*2.3*	*1.8*	2.5
α-Linolenic Acid (g)	0.2	0.24	*0.21*	*0.16*	0.25
Fiber (g)	3	3	*4*	6	6

NOTES: αT = α-tocopherol; DFE = dietary folate equivalent; g = gram; mg = milligram; RAE = retinol activity equivalent; SNDA-III = third School Nutrition Dietary Assessment study; μg = microgram. Italic font indicates values that do not meet the Nutrient Targets. Bold font indicates values that exceed the maximum Nutrient Target.

[a]The menus reported in SNDA-III had been developed using the existing Nutrition Standards (covering only eight nutrients), the nutrient values of which are lower than those of the recommended Nutrient Targets. 109 schools provided the menus for breakfast, 126 for lunch.

[b]Representative baseline menus were chosen from menus available in SNDA-III, using the process described in the section "Testing of Revisions of Standards for Menu Planning" in Chapter 5, but the nutrient values of those menus were calculated by the committee. *N* = 5 menus.

Lunch				
Content Based on *As Offered* Menu Plans				
SNDA-III Mean[a]*	Rep. Baseline Menu[b]*	Modified Baseline Menu[c]	Sample Menus[d]	Nutrient Targets[f]
816	757	592	640	600–700
10	10.0	5.9	5.9	
10.9	11.9	8.9	8.3	< 10
32	30	33	*31*	32
300	369	301	401	241
34	33	31	43	30
2.8	2.7	*2.5*	*2.9*	4.0
0.6	0.57	*0.46*	0.49	0.47
1.0	0.91	0.84	0.85	0.61
7.0	6.0	6.9	6.5	6.0
0.6	0.62	0.63	0.65	0.54
180	196	*117*	*153*	169
2.0	1.7	2.1	1.9	1.3
5.0	4.9	*4.2*	*4.4*	5.2
110	109	126	123	98
4.2	4.0	4.8	4.3	3.7
549	532	478	517	440
606	589	608	618	538
1,249	1,296	*1,228*	*1,300*	1,523
1,520	1,602	**1,558**	**1,593**	≤ 710
7.0	6.5	4.5	5.2	3.6
0.8	0.93	0.45	0.52	0.36
8	6	10	9	9

[c]The committee developed the modified baseline menus by revising the representative baseline menus to meet the recommended standards for menu planning, while keeping the adjustments to a minimum. $N = 5$ menus.

[d]The committee developed the sample menus to meet the recommended standards for menu planning and to illustrate a number of different types of menus. $N = 20$ breakfast menus and 20 lunch menus for each age-grade group.

[e]Targets based on 21.5 percent of the daily School Meal-Target Median Intake (School Meal-TMI) for age-grade group.

[f]Targets based on 32 percent of the daily School Meal-TMI for the age-grade group.

SOURCE: *USDA/FNS, 2007a.

TABLE 9-3 Comparison of Nutrient Values for Menus from SNDA-III Dietary Data and from Menus Planned by the Committee with Recommended Nutrient Targets for the National School Breakfast and Lunch Programs, High School (children ages 14–18 years)

	Breakfast				
	Content Based on *As Offered* Menu Plans				
Nutrient (unit)	SNDA-III Mean[a]*	Rep. Baseline Menu[b]*	Modified Baseline Menu[c]	Sample Menus[d]	Nutrient Targets[e]
Calories (kcal)	519	513	574	567	450–600
Saturated Fat (g)	5	4.9	3.5	4.3	
Saturated Fat (% of kcal)	9.3	8.6	5.4	6.8	< 10
Protein (g)	17	15	26	24	22
Vitamin A (μg RAE)	256	256	266	265	186
Vitamin C (mg)	37	35	63	42	26
Vitamin E (mg αT)	1.0	1.3	*1.2*	*1.6*	3.7
Thiamin (mg)	0.5	0.43	0.63	0.51	0.37
Riboflavin (mg)	0.9	0.78	1.09	0.99	0.45
Niacin (mg)	5.0	3.8	5.8	5.3	4.9
Vitamin B_6 (mg)	0.5	0.42	0.68	0.72	0.42
Folate (μg DFE)	179	162	221	207	138
Vitamin B_{12} (μg)	1.9	1.9	2.7	2.7	1.1
Iron (mg)	4.5	4.6	5.9	4.3	4.0
Magnesium (mg)	67	64	107	105	99
Zinc (mg)	3.1	2.3	4.3	4.3	2.9
Calcium (mg)	431	398	591	600	323
Phosphorus (mg)	427	381	589	592	384
Potassium (mg)	779	718	*1,165*	*1,105*	1,169
Sodium (mg)	686	659	**838**	**669**	≤ 500
Linoleic Acid (g)	3.0	3.4	*1.6*	*2.0*	3.0
α-Linolenic Acid (g)	0.2	0.4	*0.16*	*0.18*	0.30
Fiber (g)	3	2	*6*	*6*	7

NOTES: αT = α-tocopherol; DFE = dietary folate equivalent; g = gram; mg = milligram; RAE = retinol activity equivalent; SNDA-III = third School Nutrition Dietary Assessment study; μg = microgram. Italic font indicates values that do not meet the Nutrient Targets. Bold font indicates values that exceed the maximum Nutrient Target.

[a]The menus reported in SNDA-III had been developed using the existing Nutrition Standards (covering only eight nutrients), the nutrient values of which are lower than those of the recommended Nutrient Targets. 109 schools provided the menus for breakfast, 126 for lunch.

[b]Representative baseline menus were chosen from menus available in SNDA-III, using the process described in the section "Testing of Revisions of Standards for Menu Planning" in Chapter 5, but the nutrient values of those menus were calculated by the committee. *N* = 5 menus.

Lunch				
Content Based on *As Offered* Menu Plans				
SNDA-III Mean[a*]	Rep. Baseline Menu[b*]	Modified Baseline Menu[c]	Sample Menus[d]	Nutrient Targets[f]
857	913	845	789	750–850
10	9.2	7.1	6.8	
10.6	9.1	7.5	7.8	< 10
33	33	34	35	32
299	252	397	377	277
39	20	63	52	39
2.8	2.9	*4.7*	*3.5*	5.4
0.6	0.73	0.63	0.60	0.56
1.0	1.12	1.00	0.94	0.67
8.0	9.1	7.4	7.3	7.3
0.6	0.63	0.71	0.71	0.63
184	243	*168*	*167*	205
2.0	2.0	2.0	2.0	1.6
5.2	6.0	*5.4*	*5.2*	5.9
113	115	169	156	147
4.3	4.1	5.4	5.0	4.3
547	551	576	559	481
623	607	732	704	572
1,309	1,187	*1,549*	*1,476*	1,740
1,588	2,082	**1,988**	**1,693**	≤ 740
7.0	7.7	6.1	7.0	4.5
0.9	0.91	0.51	0.66	0.45
8	8	15	13	11

[c]The committee developed the modified baseline menus by revising the representative baseline menus to meet the recommended standards for menu planning, while keeping the adjustments to a minimum. *N* = 5 menus.

[d]The committee developed the sample menus to meet the recommended standards for menu planning and to illustrate a number of different types of menus. *N* = 20 breakfast menus and 20 lunch menus for each age-grade group.

[e]Targets based on 21.5 percent of the daily School Meal-Target Median Intake (School Meal-TMI) for age-grade group.

[f]Targets based on 32 percent of the daily School Meal-TMI for the age-grade group.

SOURCE: *USDA/FNS, 2007a.

the calories from saturated fat) was considerably lower than the percentage of schools *offering* meals that met the standard. Limiting certain options, such as entrées that are high in saturated fat, should help to reduce this problem.

Alignment with Dietary Reference Intake

Tables 9-1 through 9-3 for the three age-grade groups compare data from four groups of menus with the recommended Nutrient Targets for school meals. (As described in Chapter 3, the Nutrient Targets were derived from the DRIs.) The tables show that the menus written by the committee, which follow the recommended standards for menu planning, meet or nearly meet the Nutrient Targets in almost all cases, especially at breakfast; and many of the nutrient values are more favorable than the averages derived from menus written under the current Meal Requirements (that is, the menus used to obtain the SNDA-III means and the representative baseline menus).

For the menus written by the committee, examination of the tables illustrates a number of points:

- The amounts of protein; vitamins A, C, riboflavin, B_6, and B_{12}; magnesium; zinc; calcium; and phosphorus all compare favorably with the Nutrient Targets for both breakfast and lunch for all three age-grade groups. (Minor deviations are considered to be within the expected limits of accuracy of the data.)
- The amounts of potassium and fiber are higher than the SNDA-III mean and the amounts in the representative baseline menus. Although some of them do not meet the Nutrient Target, some of them compare very favorably (e.g., potassium values of the sample menus actually exceed the Nutrient Target for elementary and middle school breakfast).
- As expected, the amount of vitamin E was consistently below the Nutrient Target, the amount of iron was below the iron target for middle and high school lunch, amounts of linoleic and α-linolenic acid were below the breakfast target for all three age-grade groups (amounts of these fatty acids exceeded the targets at the lunch meal), and the amount of sodium consistently was above the target maximum.
- Folate values at lunch tended to be lower than in the menus based on existing standards, and they did not meet the target for middle or high school lunch. In a few cases, the contents of thiamin and niacin were slightly below the target for lunch—the deviations may be within the limits of accuracy of the data.

Based on the above analyses, it appears prudent to make gradual changes to serve more foods that are rich in vitamin E and linoleic and α-linolenic acid (such as vegetable oils; nuts, seeds, and nut butters; and whole grains). The foods that are offered for this purpose need to be affordable, well accepted, and tolerated by the students, and they need to fit within the calorie allowance. Although peanut butter is an example of a good source of vitamin E and the unsaturated fatty acids, it is a food that many school districts omit from school meals because of concerns about allergy.

Three nutrients merit special attention:

1. *Vitamin E.* Although the vitamin E content of the menus is much lower than the target values and low vitamin E intakes are reported for schoolchildren, the committee notes that no health consequences have been associated with these reported vitamin E intakes. Moreover, evidence suggests that vitamin E intakes are underestimated in survey data because of four types of measurement errors (IOM, 2000). Nonetheless, efforts to increase vitamin E intake, such as those suggested above, are warranted.

2. *Folate.* The substitution of 1 ounce of 100 percent whole wheat bread for 1 ounce of enriched white bread (which is fortified with folic acid) decreases the amount of folate by 34 μg of Dietary Folate Equivalents (DFE)[1] (but increases the amount of several other nutrients). In some of the menus, the committee substituted 2 ounces of 100 percent whole grain foods for 2 ounces of refined enriched grain foods, thus decreasing the amount of folate in the meal by approximately 70 DFE. Selecting fruits and vegetables (e.g., orange juice, spinach) that are especially rich in folate may help make up the difference.

3. *Iron for middle school and high school meals.* The use of the nutrient density Target Median Intake approach (described in Chapter 4) resulted in relatively high Nutrient Targets for iron for the middle school and high school meals. The targets were set to cover 95 percent of the most vulnerable group (the females who were assumed to be menstruating), thus taking into account those with the highest need for iron. Although some attention to the selection of iron-rich foods may be merited within the recommended standards for menu planning, the committee did not consider it necessary to make further changes in amounts specified from the meat and meat alternates group—the food group that provides the most iron—or to place extra emphasis on the richest sources of iron within that group.

[1]Value based on computing the difference between the two folate values taken from the USDA National Nutrient Database for Standard Reference, Release 21: http://www.nal.usda.gov/fnic/foodcomp/search/.

Effects of Nutrient Targets on the Nutrient Density of School Meals

By including a maximum as well as a minimum calorie level, setting the Nutrient Targets to reduce the prevalence of inadequacy, and using those targets to develop the recommended standards for menu planning, the committee's recommendations increase the density of most nutrients (that is, the amount of each nutrient per 100 calories of the school meal). The changes in nutrient density are most noticeable for nutrients that are not a part of the current Nutrition Standards, especially magnesium, zinc, potassium, and fiber. For example, even when the calorie content is lower for the modified baseline menus compared with the representative baseline menus, the magnesium content is consistently higher. Although the potassium content of the middle school modified lunch menus (1,228 mg for 592 calories) is slightly lower than that of the representative menus (1,296 for 757 calories), the nutrient density is higher: 207 mg of potassium per 100 calories (1,228 divided by 5.92) compared with 171 mg potassium per 100 calories (1,296 divided by 7.57). Even when the calorie content of a meal increases, such as for breakfast for middle school children, the nutrient density of several nutrients is increased in the modified baseline menus. For example, the potassium per 100 calories of the middle school breakfast increased from 151 to 180 mg per 100 calories. Consuming a variety of nutrient-dense foods[2] or foods rich in specific nutrients is a recurrent recommendation in the *Dietary Guidelines*. Thus, the increases in nutrient density that result from the revised standards indicate an important way in which the new standards conform to *Dietary Guidelines*. Improved nutrient density also lays a foundation for overall improvement in total daily nutrient intakes by students.

Effects of Nutrient Intakes from School Meals on Total Daily Nutrient Intakes

One objective of the recommended Nutrient Targets and thus of the recommended standards for menu planning is to improve the nutrient intake contributions from school meals relative to the total daily nutrient intake in a manner that will reduce the prevalence of inadequacy and excessive intake as defined by the DRIs. From Tables 3-2 and 3-3 in Chapter 3, it is clear that the nutrients of potential concern for at least three age-grade-gender groups include vitamins A, C, and E, folate, phosphorus, magnesium, zinc, potassium, and fiber. The age-gender group at apparently highest risk is females ages 14–18 years. However, estimating the changes in the predicted prevalence of inadequacy and excessive intakes requires information on the

[2]In the *Dietary Guidelines*, nutrient-dense foods are defined as "foods that provide substantial amounts of vitamins and minerals (micronutrients) and relatively few calories" (HHS/USDA, 2005, p. 7).

ways that intakes at non-school meals might change, under various assumptions, as a result of the implementation of the recommended Meal Requirements. The committee was unable to obtain additional analyses that would provide this information. Therefore, a research recommendation addressing this topic appears in Chapter 10.

Potential Positive Consequence for Schoolchildren's Diets

The recommended *changes* in the Meal Requirements result in menus with excellent alignment with *Dietary Guidelines for Americans*. These changes are very significant, and the potential for health benefits for schoolchildren is substantial—both in terms of the foods they may consume at school and the possibility for carry-over of healthful eating behaviors outside of school.

Potential Negative Consequences for Schoolchildren's Diets

The increase in consistency with dietary guidance raises the possibility that the recommended Meal Requirements would lead to decreased participation and thus to less favorable dietary intakes. For example, nonparticipating students might choose less nutritious à la carte foods, foods from vending machines, or foods from nearby establishments. A comprehensive implementation plan will be important to avoid this possibility.

CRITERION 2: AGE-GRADE GROUPS

Establishing Age-Grade Groups

The age-grade groups established by the committee—namely, 5–10 years (kindergarten through grade 5), 11–13 years (grades 6 through 8), and 14–18 years (grades 9 through 12)—consider the current age-gender categories used in the DRIs to the extent that they are compatible with widely used school grade configurations. Because age matches were not possible in the kindergarten through grade 5 group, weighted averages of the DRIs were used in the calculation of the Nutrient Targets.

Possible Positive Consequences

Meal service may be simplified in settings that serve children in kindergarten through grade 8 in that essentially the same standards for menu planning can be applied across that span of grades. Having the three consistent age-grade groups rather than several age-grade configurations might be beneficial at the state agency and federal level as applicable to their support for and review of school food service operations.

Possible Negative Consequences

Amounts of food offered may be too large for some of the younger elementary school children because they are more likely to have lower energy needs than the older children in the same age-grade group. The use of the *offer versus serve* (OVS) provision of the law in all elementary schools might help offset this problem by allowing the children to decline a specified number of foods.

CRITERION 3: SIMPLIFIED MENU PLANNING AND MONITORING AND STUDENT ACCEPTANCE OF SCHOOL MEALS

This criterion covers a number of topics. Student participation in school meals, which the committee's criteria do not address directly, is covered in this section because of its overall importance to school meal programs and its close linkage with student acceptance of school meals.

Menu Planning Process

The committee worked to develop the least complex approach to menu planning that would be consistent with *Dietary Guidelines*. Although the recommended standards for menu planning are not as simple as the current food-based standards, it was essential to introduce new elements to conform to *Dietary Guidelines*. The committee ruled out making recommendations for nutrient-based menu planning because there was not a practical way to do so that would cover the full array of nutrients and also ensure consistency with *Dietary Guidelines*.

Advantages

The recommended standards for menu planning provide a single, primarily food-based approach to meal planning that covers breakfast and lunch for the three age-grade groups. Once training materials and methods are developed, focusing on a single menu planning method could streamline training across school districts. Required food composition data are limited to calories, saturated fat, and sodium—each of which is readily available on nutrition facts panels or from manufacturers. The approach has a strong scientific foundation that helps ensure healthy school meals for the nation's children.

Potential Negative Consequences

The committee recognizes that the menu planning process is always a complex task, especially under any set of standards for menu planning designed to be consistent with the DRIs and the *Dietary Guidelines*. Developing food-based menu plans that also meet the specifications for calories and saturated fat, that gradually reduce the sodium content of the meals, and that are operationally realistic will present challenges for many school food service directors.

Menu planning to meet the 2005 *Dietary Guidelines* requires changing the menu-planning mindset from meeting daily minimums to achieving a healthy balance of planned food items within an appropriate meal calorie range for the week. Previously, the focus was on meeting minimum amounts (except for saturated fat), and there was considerable leeway for offering extra menu items (such as condiments) and foods high in added sugars. A challenge for menu planners who have not used the Enhanced Food-based Menu Planning Approach is having weekly amounts that cannot be evenly distributed over the school days (e.g., eight grains per week means that the menu would include options with two grains 3 days per week and only one grain the other 2 days). However, meeting the Meal Requirements is only one of many aspects of the menu planning process. Time, training, and new resource materials will be required for operators to learn the new approach to meal planning. Chapter 10 identifies measures that will aid in the implementation of new menu planning methods.

Monitoring of Meal Quality

The current method of monitoring by state agencies and the committee's suggestions for the monitoring of school meals are covered in Chapter 10. Adoption of the approaches suggested there would simplify the monitoring process and be more likely to facilitate effective implementation of the recommended Meal Requirements.

Student Acceptance of Changes in School Meals

Student acceptance of changes in school meals is correlated with student participation rates. A number of changes in the Meal Requirements could influence both. Based on information about foods commonly eaten by schoolchildren and a few reports in the literature, the committee identified as follows how it anticipates that students will *initially* accept specific menu changes.

Potential Positive Effects on Acceptance

- *More fruit at breakfast.* The committee received suggestions from students to add fruit at breakfast, to use as a "topping," for example, on cereal or yogurt (USDA, 2009).

• *Greater choice at some schools.* This could improve acceptance, especially by better meeting the needs of students with religious and cultural preferences.

Potential Negative Effects on Acceptance

• *Dark green and orange vegetables and legumes on menu each week.* Few students report eating these vegetables (USDA/FNS, 2008c). Although students in schools that have the OVS provision in effect would not be required to select those vegetables, the implementation of effective educational, marketing, and food preparation strategies could improve student acceptance of these nutritious foods (see Chapter 10).

• *More vegetables at lunch but starchy vegetables served less often.* Data from the National Health and Nutrition Examination Survey 1999–2002 (USDA/FNS, 2008c) indicate that vegetable consumption by children is very low, with the exception of potato consumption (see Chapter 3). However, the committee anticipates that parents and students will ultimately appreciate the value of nutritionally improved school meals and that, with repeated exposures and high-quality food preparation, students will learn to value the vegetable items offered. Anecdotal reports from food service supervisors and newspaper articles suggest that this outcome is likely.

• *Proposed requirements to select a fruit or vegetable for a reimbursable meal.* (see section "Options for Standards for Meals *as Selected* by Students" in Chapter 7). Currently, students in most schools operating under OVS are not required to take a fruit or vegetable. The committee anticipates that the proposed requirement will become reasonably well accepted because the student has a choice of fruits at breakfast and a choice of at least three fruit and vegetable items at lunch.

• *Milk choices limited to fat-free (plain or flavored) and plain low-fat (1 percent milk fat or less).* Currently, a majority of students consume plain milk with a fat content of 2 percent or more or flavored milk with at least 1 percent milk fat (USDA/FNS, 2008c). Although the lower fat milks may not be well accepted initially, using methods described in Chapter 10 may facilitate student acceptance. In addition, the committee anticipates that the inclusion of flavored fat-free milk among the milk options will help promote the consumption of milk by students.

• *More whole grain-rich food products, fewer refined grain products.* Data from 1999–2002 (USDA/FNS, 2008c) indicate that children's consumption of whole grains is very low (see Chapter 3). This is likely to be, in large part, a function of the availability of suitable and appetizing products, and the committee expects that the availability and acceptance of these products will increase with time.

- *Nearly all entrées, cheese, and grain products low in saturated fat.* There may be some initial negative response because most schoolchildren are accustomed to the taste and texture of foods high in saturated fat. (See also the section "Student Participation" that follows.)
- *Little to no* trans *fat in the meals.* Increasingly, *trans* fat is being greatly reduced in the food supply.
- *Fewer desserts.* Anecdotal evidence and evidence from SNDA-I (USDA/FNS, 1993) and from an early study by Dillon and Lane (1989) indicate that desserts are very popular when served.
- *Less sodium in the meals.* This is probably the most worrisome of the recommended changes, because the sodium intake of U.S. children is very much above recommended levels and most schools serve meals that are high in sodium.

Evidence Related to Acceptance of Foods with Lower Sodium Content

There is only limited evidence by which to predict the acceptance of lower-sodium products by children, especially when they are introduced gradually. It is well established that taste is one of the most important factors related to food acceptability (IFIC, 2008) and that lowering the salt (sodium chloride) content of foods has a negative impact on the taste and flavor of food (Kilcast and Angus, 2007). When people undertake a low-sodium diet, observations suggest that the immediate response is a strong dislike for the foods that are reduced in salt (Beauchamp and Engelman, 1991). Although the lower sodium diet eventually may be acceptable, especially if steps are taken to enhance the flavor of food with other ingredients such as herbs and spices, this occurs under circumstances in which the study participant (an adult) is highly motivated to continue the diet.

To the extent that there are any data for children, the observations suggest that, compared with adults, children have a higher preference for salt taste (Beauchamp and Cowart, 1987; Desor et al., 1975). Thus, children may react even more strongly than adults to reduced salt taste in foods. It is unlikely that children will be easily motivated to continue to eat foods that do not taste appealing, especially if foods that contain more salt are available. Given the importance of taste in food acceptance, rapid and noticeable reductions in the sodium content of school meals would jeopardize the success in offering meals that the students will find satisfactory. Lack of satisfaction, in turn, would increase the likelihood of a decrease in student participation in the school meal programs.

On the other hand, perceptual studies on taste show that people are generally unable to detect differences between two concentrations of a taste substance when the difference is less than 10 percent (Pfaffmann, 1971). On this basis, small reductions in sodium chloride instituted regularly, perhaps only at the beginning of the school year, may be expected to accomplish a reduction in sodium intake over time without risking a decrease in food acceptability and, in turn, student participation. Overall, the choice to move slowly but systematically in reducing sodium in school meals seems prudent.

Analysis of the sample school breakfast menus indicates that school breakfasts can be planned with sodium levels close to the recommended amounts with little change of commonly used products. (See Tables 9-1 through 9-3 for the analysis and Appendix M for the menus.) Gaining student acceptance of lower sodium lunches is more problematic and is part of the reason for setting the year 2020 as the target for achieving full implementation of the sodium recommendation (see Chapter 10).

Avoiding or Addressing Decreased Student Acceptance

Decreased student acceptance could lead to the consumption of poorer quality diets by students, either by eating less of the food that is offered or by switching from school meals to à la carte meals, food from vending machines or school stores, off-campus meals, or food from home. Over time, initial negative effects on student acceptance could become positive, given appropriate measures to encourage the acceptance of less familiar foods.

With regard to increasing whole grains and especially to reducing the sodium content of meals, the committee acknowledges the need for a gradual phase-in to accustom children to the changes in school meals and also to give the market time to respond to changes in demands (expressed as purchase specifications) from school food service directors. While caution demands that the possibility of decreased student acceptance be acknowledged, the committee is optimistic that students, teachers, and particularly parents will welcome the introduction of healthier school meals and that the ultimate impacts on acceptance and participation may actually be positive. There is no evidence on which to base a prediction of the response to lower-sodium meals when offered at school without similar changes being made outside of school. Chapter 10 addresses aspects of implementation that may foster student acceptance of the changes.

Student Participation

Because the School Breakfast Program and the National School Lunch Program offer nutritious foods that promote schoolchildren's growth, health, and readiness to learn, schools aim for high student participation rates in these programs. The available data on which to base confident predictions of any effects of the proposed changes on participation rates are limited. The committee anticipates that participation rates will be strongly affected by economic factors. It further anticipates that, overall, students and parents will value a change toward more healthful school meals.

The most promising data related to student participation rates are found in a recent empirical analysis conducted in Minnesota (Wagner et al., 2007). These investigators present preliminary evidence that lunch sales do not decline when "healthier"[3] meals are served. This finding suggests that participation rates are maintained with improvements in the nutritional quality of the meal. As described below, there is some evidence that changes toward reducing high-fat choices and increasing the availability of low-fat entrée choices in school lunch improve nutrient intakes and may increase participation in school lunch.

One intervention to increase fruit and vegetable availability in school breakfasts resulted in increased participation (Woodward-Lopez and Webb, 2008). Several evaluations of more comprehensive attempts to improve the nutritional value of school lunches—from San Francisco (Wojcicki and Heyman, 2006), Texas (Cullen et al., 2008), and California middle and high schools (Center for Weight and Health, 2006)—all have shown increases in participation.

Several studies have examined the effects of increasing the frequency of offering lower fat entrées in school lunch. Whitaker et al. (1993, 1994) worked in elementary schools in Bellevue, Washington. The initial intervention was to offer low-fat entrées more often. Although the low-fat entrées were selected less frequently than the higher fat entrées (29 percent of students selected the lower fat entrées—without any further intervention or awareness of the intervention on the part of the students), there was no effect on participation rates (Whitaker et al., 1993). In a subsequent study, the same intervention was used in a randomized design, but the study was expanded by engaging parents at a low level as agents of change. This was accomplished by providing information: menus that emphasized (by bold font) the lower fat alternative entrées, facts about the fat content of both entrées, and menu nutrition information. The results were an increase in the selection of low-fat entrées and no change in school lunch participation (Whitaker et al., 1994). In a later study in central Texas elementary schools, an intervention was introduced to offer lower fat entrées more frequently, followed by a reduction in the frequency of offering higher fat alternative entrées (Bartholomew and Jowers, 2006). In this study, the percentage of students selecting the lower fat entrée increased, and there was a 20 percent reduction in selection of the higher fat entrée. School lunch participation increased slightly overall.

[3]The scoring method described in the article relies on data obtained from the school district's nutrition review regarding how well the school met the Nutrition Standards for the eight dietary components, and it considered the average calories per meal.

Data from the SNDA-I study, collected in 1992, indicate that participation in the NSLP is less likely when the lunch that is offered contains less than 32 percent of calories from total fat (Gleason, 1995). Although that level of fat is lower than the 35 percent upper level in the recommended Nutrient Targets, it suggests that the methods used to reduce the saturated fat content of school meals, as emphasized in the committee's recommendations, could be important to maintaining student participation rates. Low-fat and fat-free milk products, for example, may not be well accepted initially.

Evaluations of salad bar programs in public schools indicate positive effects on fruit and vegetable consumption (Adams et al., 2005; Slusser et al. 2007), but they have not examined participation rates. A program introduced in 2006 in California (and subsequently discontinued because of a lack of funding) provided an increased reimbursement rate at the level of 10 cents for every breakfast served when an additional serving of fruit or vegetable was offered. For participating schools, the impact on fresh fruit and vegetable consumption was significant. Importantly, participation in school breakfast increased enough to bring about $1 million in additional federal meal reimbursement to the state (Woodward-Lopez and Webb, 2008).

Evaluations of more comprehensive changes to school meals are few, but those that are available are encouraging. In the examples that follow, community support and technical assistance contributed to the positive results. (See the section "Achieving Change" in Chapter 10 regarding the importance of these factors.) The San Francisco Unified School District first piloted new nutrition standards for school lunch in one large middle school in 2002–2003. Then, upon finding that revenues increased, the district scaled the changes up to include the entire district the following year (Wojcicki and Heyman, 2006). In this situation, the overall student participation in the lunch program increased in the academic year following implementation of the new standards. In total, 40 middle and high schools (almost all of those in the district) were included in the evaluation.

The second available experience is from the state of Texas, where a statewide Public School Nutrition Policy was implemented in 2004. The policy incorporated a number of changes to improve the overall school nutrition offerings. An evaluation was conducted in several middle schools before and after the changed standards (Cullen et al., 2008). That study showed a substantial increase in participation from the year before the policy was implemented to 2 years following the change for all categories of school lunch (free, reduced-price, and paid meals).

In California, the pilot test of a state law that focused on the restriction of competitive foods in schools led to a more comprehensive intervention. In participating schools, the intervention included improvement of variety and quality in school meals, improvement in cafeteria environments, and the adoption of nutrition and physical activity policies. The evaluation documented an increase in participation in the meal program and a decrease in the purchase of competitive foods. The increased student participation in the school lunch program resulted in financial benefits to the schools' food service (Center for Weight and Health, 2006).

It should be noted that all the evidence cited here is from repeat cross-sectional studies and that other factors that affect participation (most importantly, factors affecting the larger economy) were not controlled. However, the available evidence shows that schools that have implemented changes similar to those recommended by this committee have experienced neutral or positive changes in participation. A caveat is that no interventions have explicitly focused on substantially reducing the sodium content of school meals. Some of the interventions, by their restriction of snack foods, would have had some impact on sodium, however.

The current economic situation in the United States has put an increasing proportion of families under economic stress. Data from SNDA-I show that students who were certified to be eligible for free or reduced-price meals had higher participation rates than noncertified students (Gleason, 1995). Since that time, the certification process has been simplified, suggesting that low-income schoolchildren may be even more likely to participate. The result is that school meals (especially for those who qualify for free or reduced-price meals) are becoming an increasingly important part of the safety net for food security for families with children.

CRITERION 4: SENSITIVE TO COSTS AND ADMINISTRATIVE CONCERNS

Costs

As discussed in Chapter 8, the increases in fruits, vegetables, and whole grain-rich foods incur additional food costs. The expected increase is likely to exceed the amount that could be absorbed by school food authorities under current federal reimbursement levels, with certain exceptions as discussed in Chapter 8. Measures to help school food programs meet the *Dietary Guidelines* incur cost increases and an increased need for administrative support. An overview of strategies to control the overall cost of food service operations appears in Chapter 10, Box 10-2.

Administrative Concerns

Change always leads to administrative concerns, and the committee lists a number of potential concerns below.

Purchasing

In the short term, food service directors may face challenges in obtaining acceptable food products, especially ones that are reduced in sodium and saturated fat (and, in some areas, whole grain-rich foods). The new standards for menu planning will require greater attention to writing appropriate specifications for food processors or vendors.

Preparation and Meal Service

The committee developed the standards for menu planning with the intent of making them adaptable to many types of food service operations. The sample menus in Appendix M illustrate this point. Nonetheless, the addition of food items, namely at least one more fruit at breakfast and (for some programs) one more vegetable at lunch, will increase time and space requirements at schools that have not already taken the initiative to make these increases. Data from SNDA-III (USDA/FNS, 2007a), however, indicate that many schools already offer an additional fruit, vegetable, or both over amounts specified in the current Meal Requirements.

Equipment and Kitchen and Storeroom Space

Improving the quality of school meals by adding fruits and vegetables and decreasing saturated fat and sodium may call for additional equipment and kitchen and storeroom space in many food service operations. The extent of the need will depend on the current status and on decisions related to (1) the use of purchased entrées and ready-to-eat fruits and vegetables or (2) in-house preparation of those items. Some food service operations may need to add refrigerator or freezer space; fruit and vegetable preparation sinks; work table space; and special utensils to cut, dice, or chop fruits and vegetables for ready-to-eat portions. Some may need to replace fryers with steamers, microwave ovens, and combi ovens. To handle additional menu items, serving lines may need more refrigerated units, hot wells, and utility carts. Additional small serving and portioning equipment may be needed.

Effects on Student Participation Rates

Student participation rates are a major administrative concern because they affect revenue, as noted above, and thus are closely linked to the financial viability of school meal programs. Because of the close link of participation rates with student acceptance of school meals, the evidence concerning student participation rates was reviewed in the previous section.

SUMMARY

Apart from cost data (covered in Chapter 8), relatively little evidence is available on which to base predictions of the impact of implementing the recommended Meal Requirements for school meals. It is clear that the recommended standards for menu planning will result in menus that are much more consistent with the DRIs and the *Dietary Guidelines* than are the current standards for menu planning. In addition, the meals will provide more nutrients relative to calories, and the recommended option for meals *as selected* by the student may improve actual consumption of fruits and vegetables. In some school settings, the initial need (and therefore the cost) for equipment and/or training may be increased. The literature suggests that student acceptance can be achieved and participation rates maintained if appropriate methods are used for implementing change.

10

Implementation, Evaluation, and Research

The effectiveness of recommended Nutrient Targets and Meal Requirements will be determined in large part by the extent to which the children consume appropriate amounts of the foods that are offered and the manner in which the targets and requirements are implemented, monitored, and evaluated. *Monitoring* refers to a review of how well the revised Meal Requirements are being implemented for the purpose of quality improvement at the local level. *Evaluation* refers to well-designed studies to examine the value of the Meal Requirements in meeting overall programmatic goals. Topics covered under implementation include key elements of achieving change, menu planning, school food service program operation, technical support for school food service operators, monitoring the quality of school meals, achieving long-term goals related to reducing sodium and increasing the whole grain content of meals, and the updating of the Nutrient Targets and Meal Requirements in response to future changes in *Dietary Guidelines for Americans* and the Dietary Reference Intakes (DRIs). Specific recommendations are given related to technical support for food service workers, procedures for monitoring, and measures related to the sodium and whole grain content of prepared foods. The chapter concludes with the committee's recommendations related to evaluation and research.

IMPLEMENTATION

Achieving Change

Background

Making a substantial change in menus for the school meal programs calls for a holistic approach to the entire food service operation. A strategic plan that introduces change incrementally over a realistic time frame—one developed with the involvement of key stakeholders—is desirable. The foremost concern of all operators is the possibility that modifications may negatively affect student participation. Especially in the current economy, any loss of revenue based on decreased participation presents a real threat to the financial stability of the program. Operators are acutely aware of student preferences; they know that students often decide whether or not to eat a school meal based on what is on the menu and not on hunger alone. Thus, careful consideration needs to be given to many aspects of implementing change.

Community-level strategies that can be used to promote change include engaging the school community, peer involvement, nutrition education, parental and community involvement, the training of food service workers and the involvement of the food industry. Brief summaries of these topics appear below. Some studies illustrate measures that improve the acceptance of more healthful foods outside the school setting. For example, Garey et al. (1990), Hinkle et al. (2008), and Wechsler et al. (1998) describe strategies for increasing the acceptance of milk products with lower fat content, several of which are similar to the strategies described below. Key factors that may be beyond the school food operators' control but that influence student acceptance of the food offered include the time of the meal and the amount of time allowed for obtaining and eating the meal, the eating spaces available, the timing of recess, and access to competitive foods. "Making It Happen" (http://teamnutrition.usda.gov/resources/makingithappen.html), a joint project of USDA and Health and Human Services, is a source of locally tested ideas for improving the nutritional quality of all foods and beverages offered and sold on school campuses.

Engaging the School Community

Engaging the school community in the implementation of the new recommendations is essential. Several interventions noted the importance of formative research with the target audiences. For example, strategies that engage the school community include taste testing for the students to improve preference for new items (Fulkerson et al., 2004; Snyder et al., 1999; Wechsler et al., 1998), signage on the food line (Fulkerson et al., 2004; Wechsler et al., 1998), product positioning (Goldberg and Gunasti, 2007; Wechsler et al., 1998), posters (Fulkerson et al., 2004; Snyder et al., 1999; Wechsler et al., 1998), media campaigns (Fulkerson et al., 2004; Goldberg and Gunasti, 2007), and celebrity endorsements (Wechsler et al., 1998).

Peer Involvement

Peer involvement is another strategy for promoting recommended meal changes (Fulkerson et al., 2004; Hamdan et al., 2005). Student advisory councils or other school-based student committees can work with the food service staff in the interval before new regulations need to be implemented, as well as during early implementation. Input from parents and school staff is also helpful.

Nutrition Education

Nutrition education can promote behavior change. In a study by Suarez-Balcazar and colleagues (2007), just providing a salad bar in elementary schools did not improve student fruit or vegetable selections. However, the addition of six nutrition classes in the intervention school resulted in greater student selection of fresh fruit and an item from the salad bar than occurred in the schools that only had the salad bar. Some promotion or education around these food groups will be needed because the new recommendations increase the fruit and vegetable offerings, emphasize vegetable subgroups to be offered, require that a fruit or vegetable be selected by the student, and increase the use of whole grain-rich products.

Parental and Community Awareness and Involvement

Keeping parents and the community aware of the changes also promotes acceptance. Suggested strategies include presentations at parent meetings (Wechsler et al., 1998), newsletters (Goldberg and Gunasti, 2007), and the use of local media (Goldberg and Gunasti, 2007). Districts are encouraged to form school-community advisory committees to develop implementation time lines in advance of the new regulations. These timelines can inform planning for menu revisions, training, and budgets so that all the pieces are in place when the new regulations are released.

Training and Equipment for School Food Service Staff

Adequate training for school food service staff is also essential to successful implementation, and the staff will need access to the necessary equipment (Goldberg and Gunasti, 2007; Snyder et al., 1999). (Further information on this topic appears later in this chapter under "School Food Service Operation" and "Technical Support for School Food Service Operators.") In addition to learning the procedures to prepare the menu items, food service staff will need experiences to help them accept the new meal patterns and must be willing and able to give positive comments about the foods as the students pass through the cafeteria serving areas (Hendy, 1999; Perry et al., 2004; Schwartz, 2007). Training could include the use of step-by-step instructional materials—print, video, or web-based—and guided hands-on experiences.

Food Industry Involvement

The food industry needs to be a partner in achieving change because it is responsible for the diversity and quality of foods that are available for the school meal programs. Among the areas in which their partnership is essential are (1) producing appealing foods that are (a) lower in sodium, (b) lower in saturated fat, and (c) higher in the proportion of whole grains to refined grains; (2) identifying the whole grain content of foods on the label; and (3) producing foods in portion sizes that are compatible with the recommended standards for meal planning.

Menu Planning

Regardless of the approach to menu planning that is used, menu items must be compatible with student preferences to promote the consumption of the foods by the participants and also to promote optimum student participation. School food authorities (SFAs) can take many steps to encourage the acceptance of foods by schoolchildren. Among the key factors that relate to menu planning are variety in flavors, textures, and food choices; repeated exposure to less familiar foods; eye appeal; food combinations that go well together; foods that are easy to eat in the available time and eating space; and consideration of regional, cultural, and religious food preferences. All these factors need to be considered in conjunction with strategies to implement the recommended standards for menu planning.

Meeting Challenges Related to Implementation of the Standards for Menu Planning

The recommended standards for menu planning pose new challenges that will call for menu planners to approach their task with a clear understanding of the nutritional goals to be achieved, which are based on the 2005 *Dietary Guidelines*.

Assistance will be needed to meet a number of anticipated menu planning challenges such as the following:

- Planning within a calorie range that is different for each age-grade group;
- Counting both daily servings and weekly servings for planned menu items;
- Designing and grouping menu item choices to ensure that each student may select meals that meet the minimum amounts of each food group and subgroup during the week;
- Developing or modifying food procurement specifications and recipes to meet the calorie, saturated fat, and sodium specifications;
- Identifying food products in the marketplace that fit with the specifications for calories, saturated fat, and sodium and are also appealing to students;
- Implementing incremental menu item changes (to permit food service staff to develop the skills and abilities to produce and serve the new items successfully);
- Pre-costing menus and adjusting items as needed to stay within the targeted food cost; and
- Identifying the most cost-effective and student-accepted items.

To achieve the desired calorie range, the menu planners will need to consider differences in quantities and combinations of items offered on each menu, adjust portion sizes for the specific grade group, and modify food purchasing specifications and recipes to meet the desired calorie level provided by a serving. To meet the meal pattern for each age-grade group, the menu planners may need to give thought to designing a base menu that permits ease and clarity in counting the number and type of required fruits, vegetables, and grains. Ideally the menu planner will standardize the daily choices available for each type of menu item and will group like-item choices in a way that aids students in selecting items of each type.

The committee recognizes that menu planners will need assistance in achieving incremental changes in their menus, food specifications, and recipes. See the section "Technical Support and Monitoring to Benefit School Food Operations" for more discussion of this topic.

Using Cycle Menus as a Menu-Planning Strategy

The development of a 2- to 3-week-cycle menu that repeats itself over the school year with optional seasonal changes would offer substantial benefits in the implementation of the recommended Meal Requirements. Advantages relate to reducing the total time required for menu planning, improving student acceptability, controlling cost, and improving food service operations. Box 10-1 highlights benefits of 2- to 3-week-cycle menus.

The sample menus that the committee wrote to illustrate the application of the standards for menu planning (see Appendix M) provide ex-

BOX 10-1
Benefits of 2- to 3-Week-Cycle Menus

- One set of menus allows the operator to feature items rated as highly acceptable by the students within daily choices consistent with the standards. This contributes to student satisfaction and may result in higher rates of student participation in the school meal programs. It also may lead to the selection and consumption of more fruits and vegetables by the students.
- A 2- or 3-week-cycle menu aids the standardization and optimization of food procurement, inventory turnover, and daily production quantities—improving food service operations and helping control costs. Having a consistent inventory uses less storage space.
- Accurate usage projections can be established, enabling vendors and manufacturers to project their production schedules and needs and often resulting in better pricing.
- Delivery schedules can be easily set up and managed.
- Food service employees can use the food production history as a way of becoming more adept at production planning.
- Menu writing and costing need be done for only one cycle, with occasional market adjustments.
- Employees can enhance their skills in producing, displaying, and garnishing similar item combinations within the time allotted.
- Students and cashiers become more aware of what items must be selected to qualify for a reimbursable meal.
- Analysis for calories, saturated fat, and sodium will need to be done for only one cycle, with optional seasonal adjustments. The same is true for more extensive nutrient analysis that may be requested in connection with special diets.
- Health-care staff that work in schools become familiar with the nutrient contents of the meals, allowing easier control of diets for children with special needs (such as schoolchildren with diabetes for whom carbohydrate counts are requested).
- Only one cycle menu needs to be communicated to families with a calendar of cycle weeks.

amples of sound principles of menu planning. They were not designed to be cycle menus, however. Furthermore, they are not expected to be suitable for a particular school district without some adaptation to local food preferences, food availability, and the capabilities of the food service operation.

Variety and Choice

Operators are urged to offer students a choice of items within the food groups in the meal pattern, featuring foods known to appeal to their students. In some schools, foods that are healthy versions of popular fast foods and other familiar foods may improve student acceptance, especially if attractively prepackaged. In other schools, the Farm-to-School program and sustainable practices may foster student acceptance. Some schools provide free small samples of new items to encourage students to taste them. In many schools with limited eating space or very limited eating time (or both), the choices may need to be of suitable "grab and go," quick-to-eat foods.

Repeated Exposure

The acceptance of foods may be improved when the foods are served repeatedly (as is the case with cycle menus) and when children see their friends eat them. Birch (1987) and Birch and Marlin (1982) have documented that repeated exposures to foods (including fruits and vegetables) improve children's preference for those foods. Among sixth and seventh grade children in Norway, home accessibility of and preferences for fruits and vegetables were significant predictors of intake at the beginning of the study (Bere and Klepp, 2004). After 8 months, changes in home and school availability and preferences were related to changes in fruit and vegetable intake (Bere and Klepp, 2005). Exposure to vegetables for 14 days in the home resulted in higher preference for those vegetables among children ages 2–6 years (Wardle et al., 2003). Similar results were found for children ages 5–8 years in a school-based study that provided the vegetables in eight sessions (Wardle et al., 2003). Several additional studies indicate that availability, exposure, and preferences are related to fruit and vegetable intake (Brug et al., 2008; Cooke, 2007; Cullen et al., 2003; Neumark-Sztainer et al., 2003). Offering some less-well-accepted foods, in addition to preferred foods, provides students with the opportunity to learn to like the items.

Student Involvement

Student involvement in the development of school breakfast and lunch menus may contribute to the acceptance of school meals that are consistent with the *Dietary Guidelines*. Students currently play an increasing role in various aspects of school governance, and their presence and participation are required on Wellness Committees for a school district (P.L. 94-105). The committee received limited but thought-provoking input from students in the process of developing its recommendations and has worked to incorporate their suggestions in the final recommendations. Student suggestions included offering colorful, attractive fruits; preparing foods with "fun" shapes (elementary school), substituting low-fat cheeses for full-fat cheeses; and using fresh ingredients to reduce the sodium content of foods while retaining good flavor.

Vegetarian Options

In most school districts, some students prefer vegetarian meals or need them for religious reasons. In some schools, relatively high percentages of the students practice vegetarianism, but practices of vegetarians vary. For example, vegans exclude all animal products; lacto-ovo vegetarians exclude meat, fish, and poultry but consume dairy products and eggs; and semi-vegetarians occasionally eat meat, fish, and poultry along with dairy products and eggs (Craig and Mangels, 2009). Reasons for vegetarian practices include adherence to religious or cultural beliefs, health concerns, and concerns about animal welfare and the environment (Jabs et al., 1998; Lea and Worsley, 2002). Menu planners need to consider ways that vegetarians can be accommodated within the Meal Requirements.

Many SFAs currently include a variety of options that can accommodate vegetarian diets. The meat alternates (see listing in Appendix H, Table H-1) include soy protein products along with a variety of other options. Several manufacturers that produce meat alternates participate in Child Nutrition labeling (USDA/FNS, 2000b), which helps meal planners know how to include the products in school meals. Students who have special dietary needs are allowed to request a substitute for fluid milk, such as a fortified soy-based beverage (USDA/FNS, 2009d).

School Food Service Program Operation

Program Direction

It is essential to the success of a school food service program to have a qualified individual directing the program, especially during a period of transition. The person in charge of the program must have the education, knowledge, training, and experience to administer the entire food service operation. In particular, the complexities of a school food service program require strong skills in a wide variety of areas including nutrition, nutritional analysis, food safety, sanitation, budget, public finance, purchasing, equipment, personnel management, relevant computer applications, and communication to a wide variety of audiences. All these skills will be very helpful in implementing the recommended standards. A mentoring program can be developed to help directors obtain needed skills.

Effective implementation of changes in standards also benefits when directors keep current with food service industry trends and student preferences and have a broad knowledge of the industry as a whole, including relevant roles of the manufacturers, vendors, and distributors. Partnerships with industry representatives will be a key ingredient to the successful implementation of recommendations related to sodium, saturated fat, and whole grains. Directors will need to keep up to date on the various federal, state, and local policies and regulations and be prepared to produce the appropriate documentation as proof of adherence to all requirements.

Experience with and use of menu planning software helps ensure that menus meet the standards for calories and saturated fat and that gradual reductions in the sodium content of menus occur. More complete nutrient analyses can provide information that is useful to parents of children with special dietary needs. The ability to use software to create daily production records and other reports makes it possible to stay informed about essential areas of the operation and to make adjustments in menus and other aspects of the operation as needed.

The expertise of the School Nutrition Association (SNA) and its members is a valuable resource to all levels of the school food service business, but particularly to the directors and leaders. SNA provides excellent resources for networking, mentoring, and continuing education. The U.S. Department of Agriculture (USDA) and the National School Food Service Management Institute are among the entities that provide training and learning opportunities.

Attention to succession planning as part of a long-term strategic plan helps ensure that school districts will continue to be led by highly skilled personnel in the future. Mentoring and internship programs may introduce qualified candidates to the challenges and opportunities of the positions.

Cost

Operators have had to make adjustments for the last several years to keep up with increasing costs that were not reflected in the USDA cost study (USDA/FNS, 2008f). Because of the high percentage of free and reduced-cost meals being served in many schools, a majority of their per meal revenue for school meals is obtained from federal reimbursement. Although students qualified for reduced meals pay a portion of their meal costs, the total amount received per meal by the school is capped at the free reimbursement level. Thus, only the total amount of revenue for each full paid meal is under the control of the school district. Some additional per meal revenue may be received from a state, however the level of funding and criteria for receiving state funds varies substantially among the states. Thus, many school food service operations have also subsidized program revenue with à la carte or catering sales. In many schools during the past few years, these combined sources of revenue many not have been adequate to support the meal programs, so they are now operating at a loss. An increase in cost of even a few cents per meal may threaten the financial viability of many school meal programs. At current federal reimbursement levels, many SFAs will be unable to meet the anticipated increase in food costs associated with the recommended changes in the Meal Requirements. Moreover, in view of expected increases in all program costs (both direct and indirect costs, some of which are associated with the committee's recommendations), operators may need to strategically assess the entire operation to achieve maximum efficiency. Box 10-2 lists some of the strategies that can help control the overall cost of food service operations.

Use of USDA Foods

USDA offers USDA (commodity) foods to states for use in the National School Lunch Program.[1] Because approximately 15 to 20 percent of the food served as part of the school lunch is donated USDA food (USDA/FNS, 2008a), these foods have an important influence on the quality and cost of school meals (see section "USDA Foods" in Chapter 8). The Commodity Program has made substantial improvements in its offerings in recent years to become better aligned with *Dietary Guidelines for Americans* and to be more responsive to its "customers."

Types of USDA Foods Offered USDA offers both perishable and nonperishable products. The major types of foods are red meat, fish, poultry, egg products, fruits, vegetables, grains, peanut products, dairy products, and oils. Many of the perishable products are available in a processed form (e.g., fruits and vegetables may be fresh, canned, or frozen) (USDA/FNS, 2008h).

Most of the foods offered are purchased by USDA in the category called *entitlement purchases* (USDA/FNS, 2008a). USDA makes entitlement purchases based on nutritional and customer considerations. *Bonus purchases* by USDA relate to the purchase of surplus supplies of perishable foods and thus vary greatly from year to year with regard to both the type of food

[1]The term *offers* applies because neither states nor school food service operations are required to use any of the foods. The foods may be used in the School Breakfast Program as well.

BOX 10-2
Strategies to Help Control the Cost of Food Service Operations

- Strategically assess all areas of the operation for processes that may be outdated or that can be streamlined.
- Make data-driven decisions. Data on student participation, food cost, labor cost, equipment replacement cost, and training cost are needed to guide the operation in a strategic planning process.
- Use computer hardware and software to assist in putting processes in place (e.g., production records).
- Form a purchasing cooperative to maximize volume buying.
- Use cycle menus throughout the year to streamline menu planning and costing and to offer valid usage numbers to vendors and suppliers to obtain better pricing.
- Plan for the incorporation of the wide variety of healthy USDA foods (see "Use of USDA Foods") into the cycle menu, thus capturing the maximum amount of the district's entitlement allocation.
- Perform a cost-benefit analysis before making any major decisions such as those related to the purchase of equipment or a change to or from the use of highly processed foods.
- Make use of the local and national School Nutrition Association to brainstorm ideas and share methods.
- Ask employees to present new ideas and processes for daily tasks, and reward innovation.
- Conduct job safety analyses to reduce injuries and absenteeism.
- Create benchmarks for the organization and make team decisions based on the goals.
- Market the school meal programs to encourage student participation.
- Importantly, all the benefits of a 2- to 3-week-cycle that were listed previously increase operational efficiency. The more closely daily food production quantities match actual usage, the less waste in both food and staff time. These operational savings are essential to maximizing the percentage of revenue available to cover the higher raw food costs associated with offering more fruits, vegetables, and whole grain-rich foods.

and the amount available. In school year (SY) 2008, the bonus commodities included several fruits that were provided in canned or frozen form.

Working in conjunction with USDA, the Department of Defense Fresh Fruit and Vegetable Program (DOD Fresh Program) has made a wide variety of types of fresh produce available to many school districts across the United States. The DOD Fresh Program has increased the availability of fresh fruits and vegetables in schools, especially in schools with the highest proportion of children eligible for free or reduced-price school meals. However, because the Department of Defense has found it necessary to restructure its operations and involve commercial distributors, the program is in a period of transition (FRAC, 2008; USDA/FNS, 2008a).

Processing Processing is an integral part of the Commodity Program—about half of all USDA foods are diverted to processing. Its purpose is to produce end products that are more usable by schools. To obtain a food processing contract, companies must agree to use USDA foods according to strict specifications. For example, they might use three USDA foods (tomato sauce, whole wheat flour, and low-fat cheese) in the manufacturing of pizza with a specified nutrient profile. Advantages of processed USDA foods include the (1) reduction of (a) labor costs, (b) other production costs, (c) storage requirements and costs, and (d) some food safety concerns; and (2) the availability of foods that the school would not have the capacity to prepare.

Important Changes in Food Offerings The Food and Nutrition Service has introduced a variety of changes in USDA food offerings to improve alignment with the 2005 *Dietary Guidelines for Americans*, as summarized in Box 10-3. Several of the prepared meat and meat alternate offerings (e.g., beef sloppy joe [A716], beef taco filling [A714], cooked beef patty [A706], and frozen breaded chicken pieces [A526]) provide 5 to 6 g of saturated fat per serving (USDA/FNS, 2008h). (Serving sizes differ for these products.) Much effort is being placed on testing new products for acceptability by food service operators and students in the schools (C. McCullough, http://www.iom.edu/Activities/Nutrition/SchoolMeals/2009-JAN-28.aspx).

Barriers to the Effective Use of USDA Foods State agencies serve as intermediaries between the SFAs and USDA in the procurement of USDA foods. Known as distributing agencies, the state agencies vary widely in operation (FRAC, 2008). In some cases, state policy and procurement stifle local efforts. For a variety of reasons, not all SFAs use USDA foods to maximum advantage (CFPA, 2008; FRAC, 2008). In response to criticisms of the entire commodity system (ordering, processing, delivery, etc.), in 1998 USDA's Commodity Improvement Council requested a major project to find solutions to the identified problems. The USDA Commodity Program is now in transition and moving toward a system that will place more responsibility on the school districts and decrease the occurrence of unilateral state agency determinations on what foods to make available to the SFAs.

Technical Support and Monitoring to Benefit School Food Operations

According to the *Healthy Meals for Healthy Americans Act* (P.L. 103-448, Section 106(b)), USDA is to provide various types of assistance to

BOX 10-3
Examples of USDA Food Offerings that Are Consistent with Selected 2005 *Dietary Guidelines for Americans*

Low in Saturated Fat, trans *Fat, Total Fat, or All Three*

- Lean meat offerings include beef patties with 10 percent fat, processed poultry products with less skin and fat, 97 percent fat-free ham, 95 percent fat-free turkey ham, and turkey taco filling.
- Low-fat, reduced-fat, and lite cheeses and cheeses made from skim/fat-free milk are offered.
- No butter or shortening is offered.
- Frozen potato products must be *trans*-fat free.

Reduced in Sodium

- Chicken fajita strips have been reduced in sodium by 30 percent.
- Canned vegetables with no more than 480 mg of sodium per serving are offered.
- Low-sodium canned dried bean and canned tomato products are new products.
- Frozen salt-free vegetables continue to be available.

Reduced in Added Sugars

- Unsweetened applesauce is a new product.
- Canned fruits must be packed in light syrup, water, or natural juices.

Whole Grain

- Whole grains are available for further processing: whole wheat flour, brown rice, rolled oats, whole grain dry kernel corn.
- Whole grain spaghetti, rotini, and parboiled brown rice are offered.

Fruits and Vegetables

- The amount available increased by about 64 percent between 1995 and 2007.
- A partnership with the Department of Defense has provided fresh fruits and vegetables to 47 states, Puerto Rico, the Virgin Islands, and Guam.

SOURCE: USDA/FNS, 2008a.

schools related to the implementation of school meal programs. The listing includes "standardized recipes, menu cycles, and food product specification and preparation techniques" and information related to menu planning approaches.[2] The new recommendations involve some major shifts in the approach to menu planning regardless of the approach currently being used

[2]The law lists nutrient standard menu planning, assisted nutrient standard menu planning, and food-based menu systems; and other approaches, as determined by the Secretary.

by an SFA. Thus, operators will need to be provided with specific strategies for meeting the recommended Meal Requirements.

> **Recommendation 4.[3] The Food and Nutrition Service, working together with state agencies, professional organizations, and industry, should provide extensive support to enable food service operators to adapt to the many changes required by revised Meal Requirements. The types of support required include the following:**
>
> **a. Technical assistance for developing and continuously improving menus, ordering appropriate foods (including the writing of specifications), and controlling costs while maintaining quality.**
>
> **b. New procedures for monitoring the quality of school meals that (1) focus on meeting relevant *Dietary Guidelines* and (2) provide information for continuous quality improvement and for mentoring food service workers to assist in performance improvement.**

Technical Support

To facilitate effective implementation of the recommended standards for menu planning, planners may need many forms of technical support. The earlier section "Menu Planning" identifies many of the areas in which technical assistance will be needed. One priority is collaboration with school food service directors to revise related menu planning guidance materials, including the *Food Buying Guide for Child Nutrition Programs* (USDA/FNS, 2009c) to make its content compatible with the recommended Meal Requirements. The committee encourages the simplification of procedures for selecting specific foods in amounts that will meet the standards. Emphasis should be placed on assisting operators to follow the meal patterns while keeping calories within the minimum and maximum levels, keeping saturated fat content below the maximum, and reducing sodium content. Many of the food items offered by some schools contain more solid fat or calories (often from high-fat entrées or bread products, added sugars, or both) than would be compatible with the recommended meal patterns.

As example of a potentially useful approach, the committee developed a prototype of a menu checking tool (see Appendix Table M-7), which might be developed further and tested in a variety of types of food service operations. The concept is that operators would use the tool to help in menu planning, either as a spreadsheet on the computer with formulas entered to automatically total amounts or by hand entry with simple counting. Once the daily values have been entered, the formulas in the spreadsheet option would automatically calculate average calories, sodium, and percentage of

[3]Recommendations 1–3 are located in Chapter 7.

saturated fat over the 5-day week; and the spreadsheet would show how those values compare to the recommended specifications. Such a tool would provide a way to track the types of vegetables and grains that are offered and confirm that the menu pattern over the week meets the recommended standards. By entering the components, the operator would be able to identify shortfalls or overages that need correction to meet the recommended standards for menu planning.

Other important forms of technical support include guidance on the effective incorporation of USDA foods based on the new standards for menu planning; guidance on the use of production records to improve menu planning and monitor performance; and additional training and technical resources on topics such as food composition, applying nutrition and food behavior research to facilitate change, modifying standardized recipes, developing healthy cooking techniques, interpreting food labels, and developing food specifications for procuring healthier products.

Monitoring the Quality of School Meals

Because the committee determined that the Nutrient Targets are not appropriate for the monitoring of school meals, it considered elements of new approaches to monitoring. This section provides background information on the current approach to monitoring and then outlines possible elements of a two-stage approach: one targeted toward facilitating the transition to the new Meal Requirements and the second toward maintaining or achieving further improvements in quality.

Background Currently, federal regulations require that state agencies conduct two different reviews of each SFA once every 5 years. This includes Coordinated Review Effort (CRE) reviews and School Meal Initiative (SMI) reviews. The goals of CRE reviews are to determine if (1) free and reduced-price meal benefits are provided in accordance with the regulations, (2) proper meal counts are being taken at the point of service, and (3) complete reimbursable meals are being offered. Goals of SMI reviews are to ensure that (1) program meals meet the (current) Nutrition Standards and (2) SFAs receive the technical assistance and resources needed to meet the (current) Nutrition Standards. States may conduct CRE and SMI reviews independently, in any order, or concurrently. Many do so concurrently.

Under the current monitoring system, the SMI review is the mechanism used to monitor the quality of school meals. Each review covers a specific 5-day school week. During an SMI review, state agency staff members review menus, production records, standardized recipes, and nutrition facts and/or Child Nutrition labels. In addition, for schools that use nutrient-based menu planning, they review the nutrient analysis report for the specified week.

For schools that use food-based meal planning systems, the state agency completes a nutrient analysis. Results of the nutrient analysis are compared to nutrient standards and, depending on the results, state agency staff may make suggestions and/or assist SFA staff members in developing a Corrective Action Plan (CAP) to improve compliance with nutrient standards.

Current regulations require that, unless a waiver has been granted, the nutrient analysis evaluated during the SMI review be a *weighted* analysis. A *weighted* analysis incorporates data on how frequently each menu item was selected by students. These results are interpreted as representing the average nutrients in meals selected by students (*as served*). Many schools have had difficulty maintaining production records that are detailed enough to provide the data needed for a weighted nutrient analysis, especially if they offered food à la carte (not as part of reimbursable school meals) (Crepinsek et al., 2009).

In recent years, considerable attention has been focused on the CRE reviews because of concerns about improper payments made to SFAs because of errors in meal counting and claiming. The Access, Participation, Eligibility, and Certification Study (APEC) estimated that approximately $860 million in improper payments occurred during school year 2005–2006 (USDA/FNS, 2007c). Meal counting errors can occur because the planned menu does not meet the established Meal Requirements, a student's specific meal selection does not include all the components required for a reimbursable meal, or a cashier incorrectly records the student's categorical eligibility (that is, free, reduced price, or paid).

Possible New Approaches to the Monitoring of School Meals USDA could consider both a short-term approach to monitoring during the initial stage of implementation of the new Meal Requirements and a revised approach during the second stage, once implementation is well established. Both approaches would move away from the current emphasis on completing the detailed nutrient analysis and documenting compliance. The initial approach might address fewer elements at a time but occur on a more frequent basis.

During the first stage, at least for the next several years, monitoring would be directed toward facilitating the transition to the new Meal Requirements. The emphasis would be on examining progress in meeting the standards, especially those related to fruits, vegetables, whole grain-rich foods, calories, saturated fat, and sodium; identifying training needs for school food service operators; and providing needed technical assistance to improve the school meals (see the previous section for the types of technical assistance likely to be needed).

The subsequent approach to monitoring (the second stage) would continue to focus on gathering and using information to enhance the ability of food service operators to plan and offer meals that are consistent with the new Meal Requirements. Focusing on the Meal Requirements rather than the Nutrient Targets in planning and assessing school meals fits with the goals of both CRE and SMI reviews. This second stage of monitoring would focus on documenting that planned menus are consistent with the recommended meal pattern (the first step in ensuring that meals that are counted or claimed for reimbursement are consistent with program requirements). The committee is aware that, in response to the APEC study mentioned above, USDA is currently working with the National Food Service Management Institute to develop technical assistance materials related to planning and recognizing reimbursable meals (GAO, 2009). These materials are intended to help food service staff members develop approaches to make it easier for students to choose a reimbursable meal and for cashiers to confirm that a reimbursable meal has been selected.

During both stages of monitoring, a variety of methods could be used to monitor how well the program has implemented the new Meal Requirements. For example, monitors could focus on whether schools are offering only low-fat and fat-free milks, at least half of the grains as whole grain-rich products, and the required numbers and types of fruits and vegetables. This level of review could include more than a single week's menu; perhaps a full 2- or 3-week cycle. To address Meal Requirements for saturated fat and sodium, monitors could review, for a randomly selected week, nutrition facts labels for commercially prepared items (such as entrées and muffins) to ensure that the saturated fat and sodium content are consistent with targets established in a revised food buying guide. In addition, monitors could examine food production records to obtain information on the average number of fruit, vegetable, and whole grain servings being taken in reimbursable meals. This would involve calculating the total fruit (or vegetable or whole grain) servings divided by the total number of reimbursable meals.

All this information could be used to (1) establish a baseline for each SFA, (2) identify technical assistance needs, (3) prepare a plan, in cooperation with SFA staff, for addressing these needs, and (4) monitor progress over time. In addition to focusing on planned menus, the assessment would include a focus on children's selection of vegetables, fruits, and whole grains, so that these patterns can be monitored over time.

Achieving Long-Term Goals

Two recommendations are made to promote the achievement of long-term goals related to reducing the sodium and increasing the proportion of whole grains in school meals, as presented below.

Meeting the Sodium Standard and Whole Grain-Rich Food Specifications

Recommendation 5. USDA should work cooperatively with Health and Human Services, the food industry, professional organizations, state agencies, advocacy groups, and parents to develop strategies and incentives to reduce the sodium content of prepared foods and to increase the availability of whole grain-rich products while maintaining acceptable palatability, cost, and safety.

The committee set the year 2020 as the goal for achieving the recommendations for sodium in school meals—sodium values that are based on the Tolerable Upper Intake Level by age-grade group (≤ 430 to ≤ 470 mg sodium for breakfast and ≤ 640 to ≤ 740 mg sodium for lunch). This is consistent with the limited data to indicate that small reductions in taste changes are undetected (Pfaffmann, 1971) and the conclusion that gradual stepwise reductions over time may be the most successful approach. Furthermore, it is unrealistic to expect that school food operators can immediately make substantial reductions in the sodium content of school meals given the amount of sodium in foods in school meals and in the market at this time. They may need time to develop acceptable recipes that are lower in sodium, and the food industry will need time to develop the technologies to offer acceptable food products with lower sodium content.

Information in the third School Nutrition Dietary Assessment study (SNDA-III) (USDA/FNS, 2007a) indicates that the amount of sodium in school lunch meals *as offered* was 1,377–1,580 mg. Student sodium consumption from meals was about 1,000 to 1,300 mg per lunch.

Reducing the intake of sodium has been the focus of *Dietary Guidelines for Americans* and of other national health initiatives; and they have directed most attention to the sodium that is provided by salt (sodium chloride) added in processing, cooking, and at the table. Efforts to reduce sodium intake have met with limited success. In fact, given the considerable challenges associated with these efforts in the United States, the Institute of Medicine is currently conducting a study to determine strategies for reducing intakes of sodium among Americans.[4]

Salt has a unique combination of properties that may affect the texture, safety, and shelf life of many food products—as well as their taste. Thus, the use of salt is a long-established and widespread practice for products such as breads, cheeses, and cured meats (Hutton, 2002). Other ingredients may fulfill some, but not all, of the functions of salt. Furthermore, other sodium-containing substances may serve important functions in foods, including extending their shelf life and retarding the growth of harmful organisms.

[4]See http://www.iom.edu/SodiumStrategies.

Limited available information (Beauchamp and Engelman, 1991) reveals that when people undertake a low-sodium diet they do not initially find it palatable. Over time, however, the lower sodium diet becomes more acceptable. Questions that remain are how long sensory preferences persist, whether the degree of saltiness preferred increases if other high-sodium foods are consumed, whether consumers can readily accept lower-sodium single food items or meals if the overall total dietary sodium intake is not reduced significantly, and to what extent knowledge concerning adults' sodium preferences is applicable to children (Beauchamp and Engelman, 1991).

Attempts to reduce the sodium content of foods labeled "healthy" provide perspective on the challenge. In this example, the Food and Drug Administration proposed a two-tier process for defining and gradually reducing the sodium criterion for the use of the implied nutrient content claim "healthy" and its derivatives (e.g., "health" and "healthful") on individual foods and on meal and main dish products. Despite publishing a final rule (59 FR 24232) with the specifications that appear in Table 10-1, the second-tier criteria were first stayed (enforcement was postponed to a later date) in response to numerous negative public comments. Then, in 2005, the second-tier criteria were dropped in response to comments documenting the substantial technical difficulties in finding suitable alternatives for sodium that would also be acceptable to consumers. (See Appendix Q for a brief history.)

Currently, many of the popular items (entrées, cheese, salad dressings, and dips) in school meals provide between 250 and 900 mg of sodium per serving. Therefore, keeping the sodium content of school meals (especially lunch) below the maximum recommended in Chapter 7 would require substantial reductions in sodium in the foods available to schools. Chapter 7 identifies some resources that describe initial steps that could

TABLE 10-1 Sodium Criteria in the Final Rule (September 29, 2005; 59 FR 24232) to Define the Term "Healthy" as an Implied Nutrient Content Claim Under Section 403(r) of the *Federal Food, Drug, and Cosmetic Act*, 1944

	Sodium Criterion (in mg) Before January 1, 1998 (first tier)	Sodium Criterion (in mg) After January 1, 1998 (second tier)
Individual Foods	≤ 480	≤ 360
Meal and Main Dish Products	≤ 600	≤ 480

NOTE: Sodium content is per reference amount customarily consumed, per labeled serving (serving size listed in the nutrition information panel of the packaged product); and, if the reference amount is small (i.e., 30 grams [g] or less or 2 tablespoons or less), per 50 g.

reduce the sodium content of school meals by perhaps 10 percent. However, these steps would result in reductions that are substantially less than those needed to meet the sodium target.

Various types of foods (some commercial products, USDA foods, and foods prepared by the school or school district) will require reformulation. As described in Chapter 6, if a school district elects to prepare a greater proportion of the food for school meals rather than buying commercially pre-prepared products, time will be required to develop the capacity to do so. To ensure student acceptance of lower sodium foods, the process for the development and/or for the reformulation of the foods needs to include input from SFAs and students.

The sponsor asked the committee (see Appendix C) to consider a recommendation that would allow for a gradual reduction of sodium levels in school meals to meet a new standard without adversely affecting student participation in school meals and to allow time for food products to be reformulated with lower sodium levels. Based on the FDA's experiences (mentioned above), substantial technological challenges facing the food industry and school food operators, and lack of data relevant to achieving student acceptance of lower sodium foods in schools, the committee has set a 10-year window (by the year 2020) for achieving the sodium recommendation.

To ensure that action is taken to reduce the sodium content of school meals in a stepwise manner over the 10-year period while maintaining student participation rates, the committee suggests the setting of intermediate targets for each 2-year interval and the development of incentives for action. This stepwise approach is also consistent with the available data, suggesting that acceptance of diets with lower sodium content is more successful if carried out gradually as opposed to making radical reductions within short time frames. A reasonable *immediate* target would be to provide less than the mean sodium content of meals as reported in SNDA-III (Crepinsek et al., 2009). With this method for the elementary school lunch, for example, the immediate target would be less than 1,377 mg. A possible first intermediate target is a 10 percent reduction in the sodium content of the meals. For the elementary school lunch the value would be the SNDA-III mean for sodium minus 10 percent of the mean:

$$1{,}377 \text{ mg} - 138 \text{ mg} = 1{,}239 \text{ mg of sodium}$$

This value might be reconsidered based on information in the forthcoming Institute of Medicine report on strategies to reduce sodium. At the end of the 2-year interval, it would be appropriate to assess progress and effects of the actions on student participation rates, food cost, safety, and food service operations to determine a reasonable target for the next period.

The committee recognizes that reducing the sodium content of school meals as specified in Table 7-3 and in a way that is well accepted by students will present major challenges and may not be possible. All the elements of achieving change that were described at the beginning of this chapter will need to come into play. Nonetheless, assuming that participation in the school meal programs remains high, each reduction in the sodium content of school meals will be beneficial to the nation's children.

Whole Grain-Rich Food Specifications

The committee recognizes that using the whole grain-rich food criterion (Box 7-1 in Chapter 7) is likely to result in a whole grain intake that is somewhat lower than is recommended in *Dietary Guidelines*. Although brown rice and whole wheat tortillas are 100 percent whole grain foods, for example, many of the foods that meet the whole grain-rich food definition contain approximately 50 percent whole grain and 50 percent enriched refined grain. Setting more stringent specifications is not reasonable at this time because of current student preferences and experiences with whole grains, differences in product availability across the United States and its territories, cost, and limited information on product packaging regarding the whole grain content of food products.

Although the recommended standards for menu planning that are related to whole grains fall somewhat short of recommendations in *Dietary Guidelines*, they are a great advance over current regulations, which have no requirements for whole grains.

To achieve greater alignment with *Dietary Guidelines*, the following approach is suggested:

> Within approximately 3 years postimplementation of new Meal Requirements, it will be advisable to revise the standards for menu planning with regard to grains such that the proportion of whole grain (rather than whole grain-rich) to refined grain will exceed 50 percent. This objective may be attained by planning meals in which at least half of the grains on the menu are 100 percent whole grain products, increasing the percentage of whole grains required to qualify as a whole grain-rich food, increasing the proportion of grains served that are whole grain rich, or any combination of these. Product labeling with the whole grain content would be an important step.

Recommendation 6. The Food and Drug Administration should take action to require labeling for the whole grain content of food products.

Requiring manufacturers to provide information about the grams of whole grains provided per serving would enable operators to identify the grain products that would allow them to meet the *Dietary Guidelines* recommendation for whole grains. Voluntary action by manufacturers to provide whole grain content information for their food products might be achieved within a few years. Regulatory action would be expected to take longer.

Other steps that would help implement the long-range goal of meeting the *Dietary Guidelines* recommendation for whole grains include the following:

- Incrementally increase the ratio of whole grain-rich foods to refined grain foods in the meal patterns of the Meal Requirements (e.g., from one-half to three-fourths of the grains offered). Retaining some allowance for refined grain foods is likely to be needed to accommodate cultural and regional food preferences.
- Encourage SFAs to increase specifications for the proportion of whole grain in whole grain-rich foods when soliciting bids from commercial bakeries, food vendors, and product manufacturers. The *HealthierUS School Challenge Whole Grains Resource Guide* (USDA/FNS, 2009b) provides guidance for writing appropriate specifications for food processors or vendors. Studies indicate that schoolchildren will accept increasing proportions of whole grain in many grain products, up to approximately 70 percent of the total (Chan et al., 2008; Rosen et al., 2008). A reasonable goal would be to increase the proportion of whole grain to 65 to 70 percent of the grain in selected products within 3 years of the announcement of the final regulations for the Meal Requirements for school meals.
- When consumer acceptance of whole grains grows and label information includes the amount of whole grain in the product, revise the whole grain-rich food criterion so that grams of whole grain per ounce equivalent becomes the sole criterion; set the minimum number of grams of whole grain required for a food to be classified as a whole grain-rich food to a value greater than 8 g of whole grain per grain serving.

Updating Nutrition Standards and Meal Requirements in Response to Revisions of *Dietary Guidelines* or Dietary Reference Intakes

A revision of the *Dietary Guidelines for Americans* is expected in the year 2010, shortly after the release of this report, and at periodic intervals thereafter. Similarly, the DRIs for vitamin D and calcium currently are under review, and changes in the DRIs for various nutrients may be published over time. To keep the Nutrient Targets and Meal Requirements aligned with these key resources, periodic review is necessary, followed by revisions if needed.

If the current Nutrition Standards become Nutrient Targets, to be used only as the scientific basis for designing the standards for menu planning as part of the Meal Requirements, changes in the DRIs could be incorporated into the Nutrient Targets without the need for regulatory change, using the method described by the committee for setting the School Meal-Target Median Intakes (see Chapter 4). A higher target would be unlikely to affect the standards for menu planning because they were designed to balance nutrition, practicality, student appeal, and cost. A much lower target might open the way for relaxing those standards, however.

The committee anticipates that there will be little need for regulatory change in the Meal Requirements unless there are *major* changes in the *Dietary Guidelines* related to recommended meal patterns. The specification for saturated fat in the standards for menu planning could be tied to the *Dietary Guidelines* recommendation. That is, the regulation could state that the maximum amount of saturated fat is the percentage of calories specified by the most recent edition of the *Dietary Guidelines for Americans* (currently, less than 10 percent of total calories). If the recommended sodium intake is substantially decreased, it seems likely that the sodium specification in the standards for menu planning would be unaffected for some time: the committee's recommendation is for a decrease in the sodium content of school meals to be achieved by the year 2020.

EVALUATION AND RESEARCH

The recommended Nutrient Targets and Meal Requirements for school meal programs call for numerous changes in the foods that are offered, and potentially in the selections made by the students. Because the food and nutrient intakes of schoolchildren are likely to change, the magnitude and direction of the changes should be evaluated. The revisions to the Meal Requirements may also have an impact on student acceptance and participation rates, school food service operations, and the cost of the program. All these outcomes should be carefully evaluated after implementation of the revisions. In addition, the committee agreed that research is needed in several areas to better revise and implement the recommended Nutrient Targets and Meal Requirements in the future.

Recommendations for Evaluation

Recommendation 7. Relevant agencies in USDA and other federal departments should provide support for the conduct of studies to evaluate the revised Meal Requirements for the School Breakfast Program and the National School Lunch Program.

a. USDA should continue funding for periodic School Nutrition Dietary Assessment studies, with the intermittent addition of a cost component.

b. USDA should take the lead in providing funding to conduct well-designed short-term studies in varied school settings to better understand how the new Meal Requirements change children's total and school meal dietary intakes, student participation, food service operations, and cost.

The following sections illustrate the types of evaluations that fall under this recommendation.

Evaluation Using the School Nutrition Dietary Assessment Studies

Many of the changes resulting from the revised standards can be evaluated by the SNDA studies, and the committee urges continuation of these studies with the addition of a cost component. USDA has been funding evaluations of nutrients and costs, but in separate studies and sometimes at different points in time. The dovetailing of these efforts would allow nutrients and food groups to be examined jointly with costs. Specific questions of importance could be addressed by comparing the results of the next SNDA study with those from SNDA-III. Following are several topics of particular interest.

Nutrient Inadequacy

1. What is the effect of recommended changes in school Meal Requirements on children's nutrient intakes, both from the school meals and across the day? How did the prevalence of nutrient inadequacy change? (The Nutrient Targets would be useful in such a study.)

2. How do changes in the Meal Requirements influence nutrient intakes from other meals?

3. Some of the assumptions that are inherent in the use of the Target Median Intake method to set the Nutrient Targets are untested in a school meals setting and should be evaluated:

a. How did the changes to the school meals affect intakes in the lower tails of the distribution? For example, how did the shape of the distributions change when the mean intake was increased or decreased?

b. For nutrients with an Adequate Intake, is it appropriate to set the Target Median Intake equal to the Adequate Intake, or do the distributions of intake indicate a concern about some groups of schoolchildren with very low intakes?

Nutrient Intakes above the Tolerable Upper Intake Level

1. Do the recommended changes in the school Meal Requirements result in an increase in the prevalence of intakes above the Tolerable Upper Intake Level for any of the age-gender subgroups? If so, are strategies needed to reduce the very high intakes?

2. Did the changes to the school Meal Requirements affect intakes in the upper tails of the distribution in the same way as intakes at the mean? If not, how did the distributions change?

3. Did sodium intakes decrease so that mean intakes are closer to the Tolerable Upper Intake Level?

Achievement of Appropriate Calorie Intakes at School Meals

1. Were the desired mean calorie intakes for each age-grade group achieved?

2. How did the distribution of energy intake per kilogram of body weight change?

Achievement of Consistency with the *Dietary Guidelines*

1. How do children's food group intakes compare with the daily dietary patterns recommended by MyPyramid after the new Meal Requirements have been fully implemented for at least one year? Specifically, did consumption of fruits, vegetables, and whole grain-rich foods increase at the school meals and across the day?

2. What changes have occurred in children's food group intakes from other meals?

3. What changes have occurred in children's intake of discretionary calories, both at the school meals and throughout the day?

4. What changes have occurred in intakes of saturated fat?

Evaluation by Conducting Well-Defined, Short-Term Studies

The committee recommends that well-defined, short-term studies be conducted in a variety of settings to better understand the impact of the new Meal Requirements. These studies could address all the above measures, either separately or simultaneously, within a school or school district. A pre-post study design would be desirable, in which data on children's intakes (both at school and throughout the day), meal participation rates, school food service operations, and school meal costs are collected at two time points: (1) prior to implementation of the revised Meal Requirements and (2) after implementation, allowing for a period of transition to fully adapt to the new requirements. With this design, changes in the measures could be evaluated within the same group of children. This type of short-term study would be conducted in different age-grade groups of students (elementary school, middle school, high school) and in a variety of school settings (large, small, ethnically diverse, etc.).

Other Relevant Topics for Evaluation

In addition, the committee considers the following topics to be worthy of evaluation.

Acceptance of Meals and Participation in the Program

1. What is the effect of recommended changes in the Meal Requirements on school meal participation? Evaluate the impact on free and reduced-price participation and on paid-meal participation.
2. How does offering multiple choices of entrées, fruits, and vegetables affect student acceptance (and participation rates)?
3. What is the student acceptance of lower sodium foods?
4. What are the effects of new guidelines for the variety of vegetables to be offered?
5. What is the impact of the revised Meal Requirements under the *offer versus serve* provision of the law on student selection of vegetables and other meal components?

Challenges to School Food Service Operations

1. How do the recommended Meal Requirements affect food service operations; how can any problems be addressed?
2. To what extent have vendors responded to the changes by making recommended foods more available and in appropriate portion sizes?
3. How do the new Meal Requirements affect food waste?
4. How do the new Meal Requirements affect the ease of administration for state agencies? Are there differences across states based on foods available and ways of administering the program?

Changes to the Cost of the Programs How well do projected costs compare to the actual costs of implementing the changes, and how do costs vary by geographic location or size of the school district?

Child Health Outcomes It would also be desirable to conduct longer term studies of potential improvements in children's health as a result of the new Meal Requirements. Such studies might have a cross-sectional design (for example, comparing participants and nonparticipants after adjusting for confounding factors) or a longitudinal design (for example, tracking changes in health outcomes over time). Of particular interest are studies that could evaluate the impact of the Meal Requirements on the prevalence of childhood overweight and obesity.

Recommendations for Research

The committee asked several questions for which scientific answers were unavailable. This lack of information led to uncertainty about the potential effectiveness of some of the recommendations for Meal Requirements for school meals.

Recommendation 8. The committee recommends that agencies of USDA, of other federal departments, and relevant foundations fund research studies on topics related to the implementation of the new Meal Requirements, children's acceptance of and participation in school meals, and children's health—especially the following:

a. Effects of the recommended range of calorie levels on the adequacy of energy intakes for individual children within each of the age-grade categories.

b. Impacts of various approaches to reducing the sodium content of school meals and student acceptance of reduced-sodium foods.

c. Impacts of various approaches to increase the acceptance of whole grain-rich products.

d. Fruit and vegetable options and preparation methods that will increase consumption and decrease waste.

e. Effects on cost, waste, and food and nutrient intakes of various options to govern the number and types of foods students must accept for a reimbursable meal under the *offer versus serve* provision of the law.

f. Targeted approaches to decreasing the prevalence of nutrient inadequacy that do not require increasing the intakes of all children.

g. Changes in child health as a result of the new standards.

The full set of recommended research topics appears below.

1. To what extent do the revised calorie standards for school meals provide adequate calories for all without providing excessive calories for some? For example, the recommended minimum and maximum calorie levels were set based on the average for males and females. Does this cause "hunger" issues with males or athletes (male and female) or both, especially among older students for whom the range of caloric needs is higher? Studies are needed that measure energy intakes relative to energy needs at the individual level, as well as satiety, across different strata of family food security and incomes.

2. How can sodium levels of school meals be reduced without adversely affecting student acceptance? What is the minimum sodium content for foods (such as an entrée) to be acceptable and safe? Is a stepped reduc-

tion in sodium levels more likely to result in student acceptance of low-sodium foods? What other strategies can help to reduce the sodium content in school meals (e.g., the use of salt substitute, herbs, pairing flavors such as citrus)?

3. What are strategies for achieving high student acceptance of 100 percent whole grain products (products with 16 g or more of whole grains per 1 ounce equivalent portion)?

4. How can the recommended changes in the school meals be complemented by other programs to increase fruit and vegetable consumption? For example, what is the effect of the USDA Fresh Fruit and Vegetable Program on children's total daily intake of fruits, vegetables, and other foods? How does the provision of a fruit or vegetable snack in the morning affect lunch intake? What is the impact and cost of using salad bars?

5. To what extent can logistical strategies (such as holding recess before rather than after lunch or lengthening the lunch period) increase schoolchildren's consumption of food groups encouraged in the *Dietary Guidelines for Americans*?

6. What guidelines would improve schoolchildren's adherence to the *Dietary Guidelines* without increasing food waste? For example, what strategies would improve student selection of vegetables, particularly of dark green and orange vegetables?

7. The methods used to set the School Meal-Target Median Intakes assume it is necessary to shift the full distribution of intakes to reduce the prevalence of inadequacy, but there may be alternative methods of reducing the prevalence of inadequacy. For example, could subpopulations with the lowest intakes of nutrients be identified and specifically targeted (e.g., provide calcium-rich foods to children who avoid milk)? Such targeted approaches could reduce costs while contributing to increased nutrient intakes.

The committee notes that there are many interactions between the school meal programs and competitive foods in schools (for example, see the benchmarks in Chapter 6 [Next Steps] in *Nutrition Standards for Foods in Schools* [IOM, 2007]). Some of the benchmarks for an implementation and evaluation plan are relevant to the school meals programs.

SUMMARY

Successful implementation of the recommended Nutrient Targets and Meal Requirements will require attention to key elements of achieving change, menu planning, school food service program operation, technical support for school food service operators, monitoring of the quality of school meals, and achieving long-term goals related to reducing sodium and increasing the whole grain content of school meals. Acting on recommendations for evaluation and research will provide information needed for further improvements to standards for school meals and methods for planning intakes by groups.

11

References

Adamo, K. B., S. A. Prince, A. C. Tricco, S. Connor-Gorber, and M. Tremblay. 2009. A comparison of indirect versus direct measures for assessing physical activity in the pediatric population: A systematic review. *International Journal of Pediatric Obesity* 4(1):2–27.

Adams, M. A., R. L. Pelletier, M. M. Zive, and J. F. Sallis. 2005. Salad bars and fruit and vegetable consumption in elementary schools: A plate waste study. *Journal of the American Dietetic Association* 105(11):1789–1792.

Alston, J. M., D. A. Sumner, and S. A. Vosti. 2006. Are agricultural policies making us fat? Likely links between agricultural policies and human nutrition and obesity, and their policy implications. *Review of Agricultural Economics* 28(3):313–322.

Alston, J. M., D. A. Sumner, and S. A. Vosti. 2008. Farm subsidies and obesity in the United States: National evidence and international comparisons. *Food Policy* 33(6):470–479.

Anderson, S. E., P. Cohen, E. N. Naumova, and A. Must. 2006. Association of depression and anxiety disorders with weight change in a prospective community-based study of children followed up into adulthood. *Archives of Pediatrics and Adolescent Medicine* 160(3):285–291.

Baker, J. L., L. W. Olsen, and T. I. A. Sørensen. 2007. Childhood body-mass index and the risk of coronary heart disease in adulthood. *New England Journal of Medicine* 357(23):2329–2337.

Bartholomew, J. B., and E. M. Jowers. 2006. Increasing frequency of lower-fat entrees offered at school lunch: An environmental change strategy to increase healthful selections. *Journal of the American Dietetic Association* 106(2):248–252.

Beauchamp, G. K., and B. J. Cowart. 1987. Preference of extremely high levels of salt among young children. *Annals of the New York Academy of Sciences* 510:171–172.

Beauchamp, G. K., and K. Engelman. 1991. High salt intake. Sensory and behavioral factors. *Hypertension* 17(1 Suppl.):176–181.

Beghin, J. C., and H. H. Jensen. 2008. Farm policies and added sugars in US diets. *Food Policy* 33(6):480–488.

Bere, E., and K. I. Klepp. 2004. Correlates of fruit and vegetable intake among Norwegian schoolchildren: Parental and self-reports. *Public Health Nutrition* 7(8):991–998.

Bere, E., and K. I. Klepp. 2005. Changes in accessibility and preferences predict children's future fruit and vegetable intake. *International Journal of Behavioral Nutrition and Physical Activity* 2:15.

Birch, L. L. 1987. The role of experience in children's food acceptance patterns. *Journal of the American Dietetic Association* 87(9 Suppl.):S36–S40.

Birch, L. L., and D. W. Marlin. 1982. I don't like it; I never tried it: Effects of exposure on two-year-old children's food preferences. *Appetite* 3(4):353–360.

Briefel, R. R., and C. L. Johnson. 2004. Secular trends in dietary intake in the United States. *Annual Review of Nutrition* 24:401–431.

Briefel, R., M. K. Crepinsek, C. Cabili, A. Wilson, and P. M. Gleason. 2009. School food environments and practices affect dietary behaviors of US public school children. *Journal of the American Dietetic Association* 109(2 Suppl.):S91–S107.

Britten, P., K. Marcoe, S. Yamini, and C. Davis. 2006. Development of food intake patterns for the MyPyramid food guidance system. *Journal of Nutrition Education and Behavior* 38(6 Suppl.):S78–S92.

Brug, J., N. I. Tak, S. J. te Velde, E. Bere, and I. de Bourdeaudhuij. 2008. Taste preferences, liking and other factors related to fruit and vegetable intakes among schoolchildren: Results from observational studies. *British Journal of Nutrition* 99(Suppl. 1):S7–S14.

CDC (Centers for Disease Control and Prevention). 2002. Iron Deficiency—United States, 1999–2000. *Morbidity and Mortality Weekly Report* 51(40):897–899, http://www.cdc.gov/mmwr/preview/mmwrhtml/mm5140a1.htm (accessed October 22, 2008).

CDC. 2008. *Overweight Prevalence.* http://www.cdc.gov/obesity/childhood/prevalence.html (accessed July 23, 2009).

CDC. 2009. *Defining Childhood Overweight and Obesity.* http://www.cdc.gov/obesity/childhood/defining.html (accessed July 10, 2009).

Center for Weight and Health, University of California, Berkeley. 2006. *LEAF (Linking Education, Activity, and Food): Pilot Implementation of SB 19 in California Middle and High Schools.* Berkeley, CA: University of California, Berkeley. http://www.cnr.berkeley.edu/cwh/activities/LEAF.shtml (accessed August 19, 2009).

CFPA (California Food Policy Advocates). 2008. *The Federal Child Nutrition Commodity Program: A Report on Nutritional Quality.* Oakland, CA: CFPA. http://www.cfpa.net/School_Food/commodities_full.pdf (accessed September 29, 2008).

Chan, H. W., T. Burgess Champoux, M. Reicks, Z. Vickers, and L. Marquart. 2008. White whole-wheat flour can be partially substituted for refined-wheat flour in pizza crust in school meals without affecting consumption. *Journal of Child Nutrition and Management* 32(1), http://docs.schoolnutrition.org/newsroom/jcnm/08spring/chan/index.asp (accessed August 19, 2009).

Chumlea, W. C., C. M. Schubert, A. F. Roche, H. E. Kulin, P. A. Lee, J. H. Himes, and S. S. Sun. 2003. Age at menarche and racial comparisons in US girls. *Pediatrics* 111(1):110–113.

Cooke, L. 2007. The importance of exposure for healthy eating in childhood: A review. *Journal of Human Nutrition and Dietetics* 20(4):294–301.

Corder, K., U. Ekelund, R. M. Steele, N. J. Wareham, and S. Brage. 2008. Assessment of physical activity in youth. *Journal of Applied Physiology* 105(3):977–987.

Craig, W. J., and A. R. Mangels. 2009. Position of the American Dietetic Association: vegetarian diets. *Journal of the American Dietetic Association* 109(7):1266–1282.

Crepinsek, M. K., A. R. Gordon, P. M. McKinney, E. M. Condon, and A. Wilson. 2009. Meals offered and served in US public schools: Do they meet nutrient standards? *Journal of the American Dietetic Association* 109(2 Suppl.):S31–S43.

Cullen, K. W., T. Baranowski, E. Owens, T. Marsh, L. Rittenberry, and C. De Moor. 2003. Availability, accessibility, and preferences for fruit, 100% fruit juice, and vegetables influence children's dietary behavior. *Health Education and Behavior* 30(5):615–626.

Cullen, K. W., J. Hartstein, K. D. Reynolds, M. Vu, K. Resnicow, N. Greene, and M. A. White. 2007. Improving the school food environment: Results from a pilot study in middle schools. *Journal of the American Dietetic Association* 107(3):484–489.

Cullen, K. W., K. Watson, and I. Zakeri. 2008. Improvements in middle school student dietary intake after implementation of the Texas Public School Nutrition Policy. *American Journal of Public Health* 98(1):111–117.

Cusick, S. E., Z. Mei, D. S. Freedman, A. C. Looker, C. L. Ogden, E. Gunter, and M. E. Cogswell. 2008. Unexplained decline in the prevalence of anemia among US children and women between 1988–1994 and 1999–2002. *American Journal of Clinical Nutrition* 88(6):1611–1617.

De Ferranti, S. D., K. Gauvreau, D. S. Ludwig, J. W. Newburger, and N. Rifai. 2006. Inflammation and changes in metabolic syndrome abnormalities in US adolescents: Findings from the 1988–1994 and 1999–2000 National Health and Nutrition Examination Surveys. *Clinical Chemistry* 52(7):1325–1330.

Delk, J., and Z. Vickers. 2007. Determining a series of whole wheat difference thresholds for use in a gradual adjustment intervention to improve children's liking of whole-wheat bread rolls. *Journal of Sensory Studies* 22(6):639–652.

Desor, J. A., L. S. Greene, and O. Maller. 1975. Preferences for sweet and salty in 9 to 15 year old and adult humans. *Science* 190(4215):686–687.

Dillon, M. S., and H. W. Lane. 1989. Evaluation of the offer vs. serve option within self-serve, choice menu lunch program at the elementary school level. *Journal of the American Dietetic Association* 89(12):1780–1785.

Ebbeling, C. B., and D. S. Ludwig. 2008. Tracking pediatric obesity: An index of uncertainty? *Journal of the American Medical Association* 299(20):2442–2443.

FDA (Food and Drug Administration). 1999. *Health Claim Notification for Whole Grain Foods*. http://www.cfsan.fda.gov/~dms/flgrains.html (accessed May 14, 2009).

FDA. 2005. Food labeling: Nutrient content claims, definition of sodium levels for the term "healthy." Final rule. *Federal Register* 70(188):56828–56849.

FDA. 2008. *Food Labeling Guide*. College Park, MD: FDA. http://www.fda.gov/Food/Guidance/ComplianceRegulatoryInformation/GuidanceDocuments/FoodLabelingNutrition/FoodLabelingGuide/default.htm (accessed August 6, 2009).

Ferraro, K. F., R. J. Thorpe Jr, and J. A. Wilkinson. 2003. The life course of severe obesity: Does childhood overweight matter? *Journals of Gerontology—Series B Psychological Sciences and Social Sciences* 58(2):S110–S119.

FRAC (Food Research and Action Center). 2008. Commodity Foods and the Nutritional Quality of the National School Lunch Program: Historical Role, Current Operations, and Future Potential. Washington, DC: FRAC.

French, S. A., M. Story, and C. L. Perry. 1995. Self-esteem and obesity in children and adolescents: A literature review. *Obesity Research* 3(5):479–490.

Fulkerson, J. A., S. A. French, M. Story, H. Nelson, and P. J. Hannan. 2004. Promotions to increase lower-fat food choices among students in secondary schools: Description and outcomes of TACOS (Trying Alternative Cafeteria Options in Schools). *Public Health Nutrition* 7(5):665–674.

GAO (Government Accounting Office). 2009. *School Meal Programs: Improved Reviews, Federal Guidance, and Data Collection Needed to Address Counting and Claiming Errors*. http://gao.gov/products/GAO-09-814 (accessed September 24, 2009).

Garey, J. G., M. M. Chan, and S. R. Parlia. 1990. Effect of fat content and chocolate flavoring of milk on meal consumption and acceptability by schoolchildren. *Journal of the American Dietetic Association* 90(5):719–721.

Gleason, P. M. 1995. Participation in the National School Lunch Program and the School Breakfast Program. *American Journal of Clinical Nutrition* 61(1 Suppl.):213S–220S.

Gleason, P. M., and A. H. Dodd. 2009. School Breakfast Program but not School Lunch Program participation is associated with lower body mass index. *Journal of the American Dietetic Association* 109(2):S118–S128.

Goldberg, M. E., and K. Gunasti. 2007. Creating an environment in which youths are encouraged to eat a healthier diet. *Journal of Public Policy and Marketing* 26(2):162–181.

Greer, F. R., N. F. Krebs, R. D. Baker Jr, J. J. S. Bhatia, M. B. Heyman, F. Lifshitz, D. Blum-Kemelor, M. P. Boland, W. Dietz, V. S. Hubbard, S. J. Walker, and P. T. Kanda. 2006. Optimizing bone health and calcium intakes of infants, children, and adolescents. *Pediatrics* 117(2):578–585.

Hamdan, S., M. Story, S. A. French, J. A. Fulkerson, and H. Nelson. 2005. Perceptions of adolescents involved in promoting lower-fat foods in schools: Associations with level of involvement. *Journal of the American Dietetic Association* 105(2):247–251.

He, F. J., and G. A. MacGregor. 2006. Importance of salt in determining blood pressure in children: Meta-analysis of controlled trials. *Hypertension* 48(5):861–869.

He, F. J., N. M. Marrero, and G. A. MacGregor. 2008. Salt and blood pressure in children and adolescents. *Journal of Human Hypertension* 22(1):4–11.

Heaney, R. P., S. Abrams, B. Dawson-Hughes, A. Looker, R. Marcus, V. Matkovic, and C. Weaver. 2000. Peak bone mass. *Osteoporosis International* 11(12):985–1009.

Hendy, H. M. 1999. Comparison of five teacher actions to encourage children's new food acceptance. *Annals of Behavioral Medicine* 21(1):20–26.

HHS (U.S. Department of Health and Human Services). 2000. *Healthy People 2010: Volume II*. 2nd ed. Washington, DC: Government Printing Office. http://www.healthypeople.gov/Document/tableofcontents.htm#Volume2 (accessed October 6, 2009).

HHS/USDA (U.S. Department of Health and Human Services/U.S. Department of Agriculture). 1995. *Nutrition and Your Health: Dietary Guidelines for Americans*. 4th ed. Washington, DC: U.S. Government Printing Office. http://www.health.gov/DIETARYGUIDELINES/dga95/default.htm (accessed September 2, 2008).

HHS/USDA. 2005. *Dietary Guidelines for Americans*. 6th ed. Washington, DC: U.S. Government Printing Office. http://www.health.gov/DietaryGuidelines/dga2005/document/ (accessed July 23, 2008).

Hinkle, A. J., R. Mistry, W. J. McCarthy, and A. K. Yancey. 2008. Adapting a 1% or less milk campaign for a Hispanic/Latino population: The adelante con leche semi-descremada 1% experience. *American Journal of Health Promotion* 23(2):108–111.

Hutton, T. 2002. Sodium technological functions of salt in the manufacturing of food and drink products. *British Food Journal* 104(2):126–152.

IFIC (International Food Information Council) Foundation. 2008. 2008 Food & Health Survey: Consumer Attitudes Toward Food, Nutrition, & Health. Washington, DC: IFIC Foundation.

IOM (Institute of Medicine). 1997. *Dietary Reference Intakes for Calcium, Phosphorus, Magnesium, Vitamin D, and Fluoride*. Washington, DC: National Academy Press.

IOM. 1998. *Dietary Reference Intakes for Thiamin, Riboflavin, Niacin, Vitamin B6, Folate, Vitamin B12, Pantothenic Acid, Biotin, and Choline*. Washington, DC: National Academy Press.

IOM. 2000a. *Dietary Reference Intakes for Vitamin C, Vitamin E, Selenium, and Carotenoids*. Washington, DC: National Academy Press.

IOM. 2000b. *Dietary Reference Intakes: Applications in Dietary Assessment*. Washington, DC: National Academy Press.

IOM. 2001. *Dietary Reference Intakes for Vitamin A, Vitamin K, Arsenic, Boron, Chromium, Copper, Iodine, Iron, Manganese, Molybdenum, Nickel, Silicon, Vanadium, and Zinc*. Washington, DC: National Academy Press.

IOM. 2002/2005. *Dietary Reference Intakes for Energy, Carbohydrate, Fiber, Fat, Fatty Acids, Cholesterol, Protein, and Amino Acids.* Washington, DC: The National Academies Press.

IOM. 2003. *Dietary Reference Intakes: Applications in Dietary Planning.* Washington, DC: The National Academies Press.

IOM. 2005. *Dietary Reference Intakes for Water, Potassium, Sodium, Chloride, and Sulfate.* Washington, DC: The National Academies Press.

IOM. 2006. *Dietary Reference Intakes: The Essential Guide to Nutrient Requirements.* Washington, DC: The National Academies Press.

IOM. 2007a. *Nutrition Standards for Foods in Schools: Leading the Way Toward Healthier Youth.* Washington, DC: The National Academies Press.

IOM. 2007b. *Seafood Choices: Balancing Benefits and Risks.* Washington, DC: The National Academies Press.

IOM. 2008. *Nutrition Standards and Meal Requirements for National School Lunch and Breakfast Programs: Phase I. Proposed Approach for Recommending Revisions.* Washington, DC: The National Academies Press.

ISU (Iowa State University). 1997. *Software for Intake Distribution Estimation (PC-SIDE)*, Version 1.02. ISU, Ames.

Jabs, J., C. M. Devine, and J. Sobal. 1998. Maintaining vegetarian diets: Personal factors, social networks and environmental resources. *Canadian Journal of Dietetic Practice and Research* 59(4):183–189.

Jago, R., J. S. Harrell, R. G. McMurray, S. Edelstein, L. El Ghormli, and S. Bassin. 2006. Prevalence of abnormal lipid and blood pressure values among an ethnically diverse population of eighth-grade adolescents and screening implications. *Pediatrics* 117(6):2065–2073.

Janz, K. F., J. Witt, and L. T. Mahoney. 1995. The stability of children's physical activity as measured by accelerometry and self-report. *Medicine and Science in Sports and Exercise* 27(9):1326–1332.

Janz, K. F., T. L. Burns, and S. M. Levy. 2005. Tracking of activity and sedentary behaviors in childhood: The Iowa Bone Development Study. *American Journal of Preventive Medicine* 29(3):171–178.

Johnson, R. K., L. J. Appel, M. Brands, B. V. Howard, M. Lefevre, R. H. Lustig, F. Sacks, L. M. Steffen, and J. Wylie-Rosett. 2009. Dietary sugars intake and cardiovascular health: A scientific statement from the American Heart Association. *Circulation* 120(11):1011–1020.

Kilcast, D., and F. Angus, eds. 2007. *Reducing Salt in Foods: Practical Strategies.* Cambridge: Woodhead.

Kranz, S., D. C. Mitchell, H. Smiciklas-Wright, S. H. Huang, S. K. Kumanyika, and N. Stettler. 2009. Consumption of recommended food groups among children from medically underserved communities. *Journal of the American Dietetic Association* 109(4):702–707.

Krukowski, R. A., D. S. West, A. P. Perez, Z. Bursac, M. M. Phillips, and J. M. Raczynski. 2009. Overweight children, weight-based teasing and academic performance. *International Journal of Pediatric Obesity* 1–7.

Kuczmarski, R. J., C. L. Ogden, L. M. Grummer-Strawn, K. M. Flegal, S. S. Guo, R. Wei, Z. Mei, L. R. Curtin, A. F. Roche, and C. L. Johnson. 2000. CDC growth charts: United States. *Advance Data from Vital and Health Statistics: No. 314*:1–28, http://www.cdc.gov/nchs/data/ad/ad314.pdf (accessed July 28, 2009).

Lea, E., and A. Worsley. 2002. The cognitive contexts of beliefs about the healthiness of meat. *Public Health Nutrition* 5(1):37–45.

Lee, J. M. 2008. Why young adults hold the key to assessing the obesity epidemic in children. *Archives of Pediatrics and Adolescent Medicine* 162(7):682–687.

Marcoe, K., W. Juan, S. Yamini, A. Carlson, and P. Britten. 2006. Development of food group composites and nutrient profiles for the MyPyramid food guidance system. *Journal of Nutrition Education and Behavior* 38(6 Suppl.):S93–S107.

Martin, J. 2008. Overview of the federal child nutrition legislation. In *Managing Child Nutrition Programs: Leadership for Excellence*, 2nd ed. Edited by J. Martin and C. B. Oakley. Boston, MA: Jones and Bartlett Publishers.

McEwin, C. K., T. S. Dickinson, and D. M. Jenkins. 2003. *America's Middle Schools in the New Century: Status and Progress.* Westerville, OH: National Middle School Association. http://www.nmsa.org/portals/0/pdf/publications/On_Target/grade_config/grade_config_2.pdf.

McMurray, R. G., D. S. Ward, J. P. Elder, L. A. Lytle, P. K. Strikmiller, C. D. Baggett, and D. R. Young. 2008. Do overweight girls overreport physical activity? *American Journal of Health Behavior* 32(5):538–546.

Messiah, S. E., K. L. Arheart, B. Luke, S. E. Lipshultz, and T. L. Miller. 2008. Relationship between body mass index and metabolic syndrome risk factors among U.S. 8- to 14-year-olds, 1999 to 2002. *Journal of Pediatrics* 153(2):215–221.

Muntner, P., J. He, J. A. Cutler, R. P. Wildman, and P. K. Whelton. 2004. Trends in blood pressure among children and adolescents. *Journal of the American Medical Association* 291(17):2107–2113.

Murphy, M. M., J. S. Douglass, R. K. Johnson, and L. A. Spence. 2008. Drinking flavored or plain milk is positively associated with nutrient intake and is not associated with adverse effects on weight status in U.S. children and adolescents. *Journal of the American Dietetic Association* 108(4):631–639.

Nader, P. R., R. H. Bradley, R. M. Houts, S. L. McRitchie, and M. O'Brien. 2008. Moderate-to-vigorous physical activity from ages 9 to 15 years. *Journal of the American Medical Association* 300(3):295–305.

Neumark-Sztainer, D., M. Wall, C. Perry, and M. Story. 2003. Correlates of fruit and vegetable intake among adolescents: Findings from Project EAT. *Preventive Medicine* 37(3):198–208.

NRC (National Research Council). 1989. *Recommended Dietary Allowances.* 10th ed. Washington, DC: National Academy Press.

Ogden, C. L., M. D. Carroll, and K. M. Flegal. 2008. High body mass index for age among U.S. children and adolescents, 2003–2006. *Journal of the American Medical Association* 299(20):2401–2405.

Pappadis, S. L., and M. J. G. Somers. 2003. Hypertension in adolescents: A review of diagnosis and management. *Current Opinion in Pediatrics* 15(4):370–378.

Perry, C. L., D. B. Bishop, G. L. Taylor, M. Davis, M. Story, C. Gray, S. C. Bishop, R. A. W. Mays, L. A. Lytle, and L. Harnack. 2004. A randomized school trial of environmental strategies to encourage fruit and vegetable consumption among children. *Health Education and Behavior* 31(1):65–76.

Pfaffman, C., L.M. Bartoshuk, and D.H. McBurney. 1971. Taste psychophysics. In *Handbook of Sensory Physiology*, Vol. 4, edited by L. M. Beidler. New York: Springer Verlag. Pp. 327–343.

Pfeiffer, C. M., C. L. Johnson, R. B. Jain, E. A. Yetley, M. F. Picciano, J. I. Rader, K. D. Fisher, J. Mulinare, and J. D. Osterloh. 2007. Trends in blood folate and vitamin B-12 concentrations in the United States, 1988–2004. *American Journal of Clinical Nutrition* 86(3):718–727.

Robichaux, F., and S. Adams. 1985. Offer vs. serve foodservice in lower elementary school lunchrooms. *Journal of the American Dietetic Association* 85(7):853–854.

Rosen, R. A., L. Sadeghi, N. Schroeder, M. Reicks, and L. Marquart. 2008. Gradual incorporation of whole wheat flour into bread products for elementary school children improves whole grain intake. *Journal of Child Nutrition and Management* 32(1), http://www.schoolnutrition.org/Content.aspx?id=10584 (accessed April 22, 2009).

Sallis, J. F., and B. E. Saelens. 2000. Assessment of physical activity by self-report: Status, limitations, and future directions. *Research Quarterly for Exercise and Sport* 71(2 Suppl.):1–14.

Schwartz, M. B. 2007. The influence of a verbal prompt on school lunch fruit consumption: A pilot study. *International Journal of Behavioral Nutrition and Physical Activity* 4:6.

Slusser, W. M., W. G. Cumberland, B. L. Browdy, L. Lange, and C. Neumann. 2007. A school salad bar increases frequency of fruit and vegetable consumption among children living in low-income households. *Public Health Nutrition* 10(12):1490–1496.

Snyder, M. P., J. Anliker, L. Cunningham-Sabo, L. B. Dixon, J. Altaha, A. Chamberlain, S. Davis, M. Evans, J. Hurley, and J. L. Weber. 1999. The Pathways study: A model for lowering the fat in school meals. *American Journal of Clinical Nutrition* 69(4 Suppl.):810S–815S.

Suarez-Balcazar, Y., L. Redmond, J. Kouba, M. Hellwig, R. Davis, L. I. Martinez, and L. Jones. 2007. Introducing systems change in the schools: The case of school luncheons and vending machines. *American Journal of Community Psychology* 39(3-4):335–345.

Tanner, J. M., R. H. Whitehouse, and M. Takaishi. 1966. Standards from birth to maturity for height, weight, height velocity, and weight velocity: British children, 1965. I. *Archives of Disease in Childhood* 41(219):454–471.

Templeton, S. B., M. A. Marlette, and M. Panemangalore. 2005. Competitive foods increase the intake of energy and decrease the intake of certain nutrients by adolescents consuming school lunch. *Journal of the American Dietetic Association* 105(2):215–220.

Troiano, R. P., D. Berrigan, K. W. Dodd, L. C. Mâsse, T. Tilert, and M. McDowell. 2008. Physical activity in the United States measured by accelerometer. *Medicine and Science in Sports and Exercise* 40(1):181–188.

Troped, P. J., J. L. Wiecha, M. S. Fragala, C. E. Matthews, D. M. Finkelstein, J. Kim, and K. E. Peterson. 2007. Reliability and validity of YRBS physical activity items among middle school students. *Medicine and Science in Sports and Exercise* 39(3):416–425.

United Fresh Produce Association. 2009. *H.R.6124 The Food Conservation and Energy Act of 2008 (The 2008 Farm Bill)*. http://www.unitedfresh.org/newsviews/farm_bill (accessed October 6, 2009).

U.S. Bureau of Labor Statistics. 2008. *Consumer Price Index Database: All Urban Consumers*. http://www.bls.gov/cpi/data.htm (accessed October 6, 2009).

U.S. Department of Education. 2000. *In the Middle: Characteristics of Public Schools with a Focus on Middle Schools*. In *Report NCES 2000-312*. Washington, DC: National Center for Education Statistics. http://nces.ed.gov/pubSearch/pubsinfo.asp?pubid=2000312 (accessed September 12, 2008).

U.S. Department of Education. 2001. *Digest of Education Statistics: 2001*. Washington, DC: National Center for Education Statistics. http://nces.ed.gov/pubs2002/2002026.pdf (accessed August 3, 2009).

U.S. Department of Education. 2004. *Education for Homeless Children and Youth Program: Title VII-B of the McKinney-Vento Homeless Assistance Act, as amended by the No Child Left Behind Act of 2001 Non-Regulatory Guidance*. Washington, DC: U.S. Department of Educations. http://www.ed.gov/programs/homeless/guidance.pdf (accessed October 1, 2008).

U.S. Department of Education. 2007a. *Public Elementary and Secondary School Student Enrollment, High School Completions, and Staff from the Common Core of Data: School Year 2005–06. First Look*. In *Report NCES 2007-352*. Washington, DC: National Center for Education Statistics. http://nces.ed.gov/pubsearch/pubsinfo.asp?pubid=2007352 (accessed August 22, 2008).

U.S. Department of Education. 2007b. *Public secondary schools, by grade span, average school size, and state or jurisdiction: 2005–2006*. http://nces.ed.gov/programs/digest/d07/tables/dt07_096.asp (accessed April 23, 2009).

USDA (U.S. Department of Agriculture). 2005. *MyPyramid Food Intake Patterns*. http://www.mypyramid.gov/professionals/pdf_food_intake.html (accessed August 7, 2008).

USDA. 2008. *Inside the Pyramid*. http://www.mypyramid.gov/pyramid/index.html (accessed October 24, 2008).

USDA. 2009. *Inside the Pyramid: Tips to Help You Eat Fruits*. http://www.mypyramid.gov/pyramid/fruits_tips.html (accessed August 3, 2009).

USDA/ARS (U.S. Department of Agriculture/Agricultural Research Service). 2004. *USDA National Nutrient Database for Standard Reference, Release 17*. http://www.ars.usda.gov/Services/docs.htm?docid=5717 (accessed September 3, 2009).

USDA/ARS. 2006. *MyPyramid Equivalents Database for USDA Survey Food Codes, 1994–2002, Version 1.0*. http://www.ars.usda.gov/Services/docs.htm?docid=8503 (accessed August 8, 2008).

USDA/ARS. 2008. *USDA National Nutrient Database for Standard Reference, Release 21*. http://www.ars.usda.gov/Services/docs.htm?docid=8964 (accessed September 3, 2009).

USDA/ARS. 2009a. *What We Eat in America, NHANES 2005–2006: Usual Nutrient Intakes from Food and Water Compared to 1997 Dietary Reference Intakes for Vitamin D, Calcium, Phosphorus, and Magnesium*. Washington, DC: USDA/ARS.

USDA/ARS. 2009b. *USDA Food and Nutrient Database for Dietary Studies*. http://www.ars.usda.gov/services/docs.htm?docid=12089 (accessed August 6, 2009).

USDA/CNPP (U.S. Department of Agriculture/Center for Nutrition Policy and Promotion). 2007. *The Low-Cost, Moderate-Cost, and Liberal Food Plans, 2007*. Washington, DC: USDA/CNPP. http://www.cnpp.usda.gov/Publications/FoodPlans/MiscPubs/FoodPlans2007AdminReport.pdf (accessed July 1, 2009).

USDA/ERS (U.S. Department of Agriculture/Economic Research Service). 2003. *Importance of Child Nutrition Programs to Agriculture*. In *Food Assistance and Nutrition Research Report Number 34-12*. Washington, DC: USDA/ERS. http://www.ers.usda.gov/Publications/FANRR34/FANRR34-12/ (accessed August 19, 2009).

USDA/ERS. 2004. *Effects of Food Assistance and Nutrition Programs on Nutrition and Health: Vol. 4, Executive Summary of the Literature Review*. In *Food Assistance and Nutrition Research Report Number 19-4*. Washington, DC: USDA/ERS. http://www.ers.usda.gov/Publications/FANRR19-4/ (accessed August 18, 2008).

USDA/ERS. 2006. *Possible Implications for U.S. Agriculture From Adoption of Select Dietary Guidelines. Economic Research Report Number 31*. Washington, DC: USDA/ERS. http://www.ers.usda.gov/publications/err31/err31fm.pdf (accessed August 19, 2009).

USDA/ERS. 2008a. *The Food Assistance Landscape: FY 2007 Annual Report*. Washington, DC: USDA/ERS. http://www.ers.usda.gov/Publications/EIB6-5/ (accessed August 28, 2008).

USDA/ERS. 2008b. *The National School Lunch Program: Background, Trends, and Issues*. Washington, DC: USDA/ERS. http://www.ers.usda.gov/Publications/ERR61/ (accessed August 4, 2008).

USDA/ERS. 2009. *Loss-Adjusted Food Availability: Average Daily per Capita Servings from the U.S. Food Availability, Adjusted for Spoilage and Other Waste*. http://www.ers.usda.gov/Data/FoodConsumption/FoodGuideIndex.htm (accessed April 7, 2009).

USDA/FNS (U.S. Department of Agriculture/Food and Nutrition Service). 1976. Part 210—National School Lunch Program. *Federal Register* 41(114):23695–23696.

USDA/FNS. 1993. *The School Nutrition Dietary Assessment Study: School Food Service, Meals Offered, and Dietary Intakes.* Alexandria, VA: USDA/FNS. http://www.fns.usda.gov/OANE/MENU/Published/CNP/cnp-archive.htm (accessed August 4, 2008).

USDA/FNS. 1995. National School Lunch Program and School Breakfast Program: School Meals Initiative for healthy children: Final rule. *Federal Register* 60(113):31188–31222.

USDA/FNS. 1997. *Evaluation of the Nutrient Standard Menu Planning Demonstration: Findings from the Formative Evaluation.* Alexandria, VA: USDA/FNS. http://www.fns.usda.gov/oane/menu/Published/CNP/FILES/formev2.pdf (accessed August 6, 2008).

USDA/FNS. 1998a. *Evaluation of the Nutrient Standard Menu Planning Demonstration: Summary of Findings.* Alexandria, VA: USDA/FNS. http://www.fns.usda.gov/oane/menu/Published/CNP/FILES/nsmpdem.pdf (accessed August 6, 2008).

USDA/FNS. 1998b. *School Food Purchase Study: Final Report.* Alexandria, VA: USDA/FNS. http://www.fns.usda.gov/OANE/MENU/Published/CNP/cnp-archive.htm (accessed August 4, 2008).

USDA/FNS. 2000a. *Meal Planning in the National School Lunch Program.* Alexandria, VA: USDA/FNS. http://www.fns.usda.gov/cnd/menu/menu.planning.approaches.for.lunches.doc (accessed August 26, 2008).

USDA/FNS. 2000b. Modification of the "Vegetable Protein Products" requirements for the National School Lunch Program, School Breakfast Program, Summer Food Service Program and Child and Adult Care Food Program. *Federal Register* 65(47):12429–12442.

USDA/FNS. 2007a. *School Nutrition Dietary Assessment Study-III.* Alexandria, VA: USDA/FNS. http://www.fns.usda.gov/oane/MENU/Published/CNP/cnp.htm (accessed August 4, 2008).

USDA/FNS. 2007b. *The Road to SMI Success: A Guide for Food Service Directors.* Alexandria, VA: USDA/FNS. http://www.fns.usda.gov/tn/Resources/roadtosuccess.html (accessed August 22, 2008).

USDA/FNS. 2007c. *NSLP/SBP Access, Participation, Eligibility, and Certification Study: Erroneous Payments in the NSLP and SBP.* USDA/FNS. http://www.fns.usda.gov/ORA/menu/Published/CNP/FILES/apecvol1.pdf (accessed September 24, 2009).

USDA/FNS. 2008a. *White Paper: USDA Foods in the National School Lunch Program.* Alexandria, VA: USDA/FNS. http://www.fns.usda.gov/fdd/ppt-slides/whitepaper08-29-07.pdf (accessed April 23, 2009).

USDA/FNS. 2008b. *A Menu Planner for Healthy School Meals.* Washington, DC: USDA/FNS. http://teamnutrition.usda.gov/Resources/menuplanner.html (accessed July 24, 2009).

USDA/FNS. 2008c. *Diet Quality of American School-Age Children by School Lunch Participation Status: Data from the National Health and Nutrition Examination Survey, 1999–2004.* Alexandria, VA: USDA/FNS. http://www.fns.usda.gov/OANE/menu/published/CNP/FILES/NHANES-NSLP.pdf (accessed August 20, 2008).

USDA/FNS. 2008d. *Child Nutrition Labeling.* http://www.fns.usda.gov/cnd/cnlabeling/default.htm (accessed August 6, 2008).

USDA/FNS. 2008e. *Menu Planning in the School Breakfast Program.* Alexandria, VA: USDA/FNS. http://www.fns.usda.gov/cnd/Breakfast/Menu/sbp-planning-approaches.doc (accessed August 19, 2009).

USDA/FNS. 2008f. *School Lunch and Breakfast Cost Study-II, Final Report.* Alexandria, VA: USDA/FNS. http://www.fns.usda.gov/OANE/MENU/Published/CNP/FILES/MealCostStudy.pdf (accessed August 4, 2008).

USDA/FNS. 2008g. School Lunch and Breakfast Cost Study-II. In *Public use data file and documentation.*

USDA/FNS. 2008h. *Schools/CN Commodity Programs: All NSLP Commodity Fact Sheets.* Washington, DC: USDA/FNS. http://www.fns.usda.gov/fdd/schfacts/allfacts_rpts_bytitle.htm (accessed October 5, 2009).

USDA/FNS. 2009a. *Fact Sheets for Healthier School Meals.* http://teamnutrition.usda.gov/Resources/dgfactsheet_hsm.html (accessed July 24, 2009).

USDA/FNS. 2009b. *HealthierUS School Challenge Whole Grains Resource.* http://www.fns.usda.gov/TN/HealthierUS/wholegrainresource.pdf (accessed May 14, 2009).

USDA/FNS. 2009c. *Food Buying Guide for Child Nutrition Programs.* Alexandria, VA: USDA/FNS. http://teamnutrition.usda.gov/Resources/foodbuyingguide.html (accessed July 28, 2009).

USDA/FNS. 2009d. Fluid milk substitutions in the School Nutrition Programs. *Federal Register* 73(178):52903–52908.

USDA/FNS. 2009e. Food Distribution Program: Value of donated foods from July 1, 2009 through June 30, 2010. *Federal Register* 74(134):34303.

Wagner, B., B. Senauer, and F. C. Runge. 2007. An empirical analysis of and policy recommendations to improve the nutritional quality of school meals. *Review of Agricultural Economics* 29(4):672–688.

Wallander, J. L., W. C. Taylor, J. A. Grunbaum, F. A. Franklin, G. G. Harrison, S. H. Kelder, and M. A. Schuster. 2009. Weight status, quality of life, and self-concept in African American, Hispanic, and White fifth-grade children. *Obesity* 17(7):1363–1368.

Wardle, J., M. L. Herrera, L. Cooke, and E. L. Gibson. 2003. Modifying children's food preferences: The effects of exposure and reward on acceptance of an unfamiliar vegetable. *European Journal of Clinical Nutrition* 57(2):341–348.

WCRF/AICR (World Cancer Research Fund/American Institute for Cancer Research). 2007. *Food, Nutrition, Physical Activity, and the Prevention of Cancer: A Global Perspective.* Washington, DC: AICR. http://www.dietandcancerreport.org/?p=ER (accessed September 29, 2009).

Weaver, C. M., and R. P. Heaney. 2006. Calcium. In *Modern Nutrition in Health and Disease*, edited by M. E. Shils, M. Shike, A. C. Ross, B. Caballero and R. J. Cousins. Philadelphia, PA: Lippincott, Williams, and Wilkins.

Wechsler, H., C. E. Basch, P. Zybert, and S. Shea. 1998. Promoting the selection of low-fat milk in elementary school cafeterias in an inner-city Latino community: Evaluation of an intervention. *American Journal of Public Health* 88(3):427–433.

Weiss, R., and S. Caprio. 2005. The metabolic consequences of childhood obesity. *Best Practice and Research: Clinical Endocrinology and Metabolism* 19(3):405–419.

Whitaker, R. C., J. A. Wright, A. J. Finch, and B. M. Psaty. 1993. An environmental intervention to reduce dietary fat in school lunches. *Pediatrics* 91(6):1107–1111.

Whitaker, R. C., J. A. Wright, T. D. Koepsell, A. J. Finch, and B. M. Psaty. 1994. Randomized intervention to increase children's selection of low-fat foods in school lunches. *Journal of Pediatrics* 125(4):535–540.

Whitt-Glover, M. C., W. C. Taylor, M. F. Floyd, M. M. Yore, A. K. Yancey, and C. E. Matthews. 2009. Disparities in physical activity and sedentary behaviors among US children and adolescents: Prevalence, correlates, and intervention implications. *Journal of Public Health Policy* 30(Suppl. 1):S309–S334.

Whole Grains Council. 2007. *Whole Grain Stamp.* http://wholegrainscouncil.org/whole-grain-stamp (accessed August 5, 2009).

Wojcicki, J. M., and M. B. Heyman. 2006. Healthier choices and increased participation in a middle school lunch program: Effects of nutrition policy changes in San Francisco. *American Journal of Public Health* 96(9):1542–1547.

Woodward-Lopez, G., and K. Webb. 2008. *Evaluation of the California Fresh Start Program: Report of Findings*. Berkeley, CA: Center for Weight and Height, University of California, Berkeley. http://www.californiahealthykids.org/Pages/articles/CFSP_FINAL.pdf (accessed August 19, 2009).

Zlotkin, S. 2006. A critical assessment of the upper intake levels for infants and children. *Journal of Nutrition* 136(2):502S–506S.

Appendix A

Acronyms, Abbreviations, and Glossary

ACRONYMS AND ABBREVIATIONS

AI	Adequate Intake
AMDR	Acceptable Macronutrient Distribution Range
AMS	Agricultural Marketing Service, U.S. Department of Agriculture
ARS	Agricultural Research Service, U.S. Department of Agriculture
BMI	body mass index
CDC	Centers for Disease Control and Prevention
CFR	*Code of Federal Regulations*
CN	Child Nutrition
CNP	Child Nutrition Programs
CPI	Consumer Price Index
DASH	Dietary Approaches to Stop Hypertension
DFE	dietary folate equivalent
DGA	Dietary Guidelines for Americans
DRI	Dietary Reference Intakes
EAR	Estimated Average Requirement
EER	Estimated Energy Requirement

FAFH	food away from home
FBMP	food-based menu planning
FNDDS	Food and Nutrient Database for Dietary Studies
FNS	Food and Nutrition Service, U.S. Department of Agriculture
FR	Federal Register
FY	fiscal year
g	gram
G/B	grain/bread
HHS	U.S. Department of Health and Human Services
IOM	Institute of Medicine, The National Academies
IU	international unit
K	kindergarten
kcal	kilocalorie/calorie
mg	milligram
M/MA	meat or meat alternate
MPLH	meals per labor hour
NBMP	nutrient-based menu planning
NCHS	National Center for Health Statistics, CDC
NHANES	National Health and Nutrition Examination Survey
NSLA	National School Lunch Act
NSLP	National School Lunch Program
OVS	*offer versus serve*
oz	ounce
P.L.	Public Law
PPS	probability proportional to size
RA/RAE	retinol activity/retinol activity equivalent
RDA	Recommended Dietary Allowance
RE	retinol equivalent
REA	Recommended Energy Allowance
SBP	School Breakfast Program
SFA	school food authority
SMI	School Meals Initiative
SM-TMI	School Meals-Target Median Intake

SNDA	School Nutrition Dietary Assessment study
TMI	Target Median Intake
tsp	teaspoon
µg	microgram
UL	Tolerable Upper Intake Level
USDA	U.S. Department of Agriculture
V/F	vegetable/fruit
WIC	Special Supplemental Nutrition Program for Women, Infants, and Children

GLOSSARY

Acceptable Macronutrient Distribution Ranges The range of intakes of an energy source that is associated with a reduced risk of chronic disease yet that can provide adequate amounts of essential nutrients.

Adequate Intake A recommended average daily nutrient intake level based on observed or experimentally determined approximations or estimates of nutrient intake by a group or groups of apparently healthy people that are assumed to be adequate.

Alternate Menu Planning Approaches (Any Reasonable Approach) Under current regulations, menu planning approaches that are adopted or developed by state food authorities or state agencies and that differ from the standard approaches. The state agency should be contacted for specific details, as alternate approaches may require prior state agency review and approval.

As Offered The foods that are planned and prepared for school breakfast and school lunch. (Used in reference to the first element of the Meal Requirements.)

As Selected New terminology for the food items that the student places on his or her tray to obtain a reimbursable meal. (Used in reference to the second element of the Meal Requirements.)

As Served Current terminology for the food items that the student places on his or her tray for a reimbursable meal.

Baseline Menus See Representative baseline menus and Modified baseline menus.

Combi Oven A combination of a steamer and a convection oven.

Dietary Reference Intakes A family of nutrient reference values established by the Institute of Medicine.

Enhanced Food-Based Menu Planning Approach One of the two existing food-based menu planning approaches established by the U.S. Department of Agriculture that uses meal patterns with food items from specific food group components in specific amounts, by age-grade group, to plan meals. It is similar to the traditional food-based menu planning approach, except that it uses different age-grade groups and a different number of servings of vegetables/fruits and grains/breads.

Entrée A school lunch or breakfast menu item that is a combination of foods or a single food item offered as the main course, as defined by the menu planner. Typically, the entrée is the central focus of the meal and forms the framework around which the rest of the meal is planned.

Estimated Average Requirement The usual daily intake level that is estimated to meet the requirement of half the healthy individuals in a life-stage and gender group.

Estimated Energy Requirement For children, the estimated energy requirement represents the sum of the dietary energy intake predicted to maintain energy balance for the child's age, weight, height, and activity level plus an amount to cover normal growth and development.

Food-Based Menu Planning An approach to menu planning that is based on the types and amounts of foods to be offered.

Food Component One of five food groups that currently comprise reimbursable meals planned under a food-based menu planning approach. The five food components are meat and meat alternate, grains and breads, fruits, vegetables, and fluid milk.

Food Item (current definition) A specific food from the five food components required to be offered in school lunches under food-based menu planning approaches or one of the four food components required to be offered in school breakfasts.

Food Item (revised definition to correspond to recommendations in this report) A specific food offered in the specified portion sizes that will meet the recommended *as offered* Meal Standards. Student selection of the minimum number of the offered food items determines whether the meal is reimbursable.

Meal Patterns A term used to refer to food items under food-based menu planning approaches as specified for various age-grade groups.

Meal Requirements (current definition) The existing set of standards used to develop menus and meals so as to implement the existing Nutrition Standards. Meal Requirements may be met through either food-based menu planning approaches or nutrient-based menu planning approaches.

Meal Requirements (revised definition to correspond to recommendations in this report) A set of standards that encompasses (1) standards for menu planning (which are focused on consistency with *Dietary Guidelines* and the Nutrient Targets) and (2) standards for meals *as selected* by the student.

Menu Item (current definition) Any single food or combination of foods, except condiments, served in a meal under the nutrient-based menu planning approaches (nutrient standard menu planning and assisted nutrient standard menu planning approaches). All menu items or foods offered as part of the reimbursable meal will be counted toward meeting the Nutrition Standards.

National School Lunch Program The program under which participating schools operate a nonprofit lunch program, in accordance with 7 CFR Part 210.

Nonreimbursable Meals Meals that are served but that cannot be claimed for reimbursement in the National School Lunch Program and the School Breakfast Program, such as adult meals, à la carte meals, and second meals served to students.

Nutrient-Based Menu Planning One of two existing approaches used to implement the current Nutrition Standards. It makes use of computer software to plan menus consistent with the Nutrition Standards. As established by the U.S. Department of Agriculture, the approach includes the so-called nutrient standard approach and the assisted approach.

Nutrient Density (of foods) The amount of a specific nutrient in a food per 100 calories of that food.

Nutrient Density Target Median Intake The ratio of the gender-specific Target Median Intake to the gender-specific Estimated Energy Requirement—that is, the ratio of calorie needs to calorie requirements for a specific group.

Nutrient Targets New recommended goals for the amounts of nutrients and other dietary components to be provided by school meals *as offered*. Nutrient Targets provide the scientific basis for developing Meal Standards.

Nutrients and Other Dietary Components A term used to refer collectively to any nutrition-related substance that may be encompassed by the Nutrition Standards and Nutrient Targets. It includes protein, vitamins, minerals, calories, and substances such as fiber, cholesterol, and saturated fat.

Nutrition Standards The current collective term for the nutrition goals for school meals; it encompasses nutrients and other dietary components (including food categories) that are required as well as those that are recommended.

Offer Versus Serve By law, a provision that allows the student to decline a specified number of food items while still having the meal qualify for reimbursement. For lunch, *offer versus serve* is required in high school but is optional in middle and elementary schools. *Offer versus serve* is optional in all grades for breakfast.

Recommended Dietary Allowances The average daily dietary nutrient intake level that is sufficient to meet the nutrient requirements of nearly all (97–98 percent) healthy individuals in a particular life-stage and gender group.

Reimbursable Meal A school meal that (1) meets the standards set by the U.S. Department of Agriculture, (2) is served to an eligible student, and (3) is priced as an entire meal rather than priced on the basis of individual items. Such meals qualify for reimbursement with federal funds.

Representative Baseline Menus Menus from the third School Nutrition Dietary Assessment study that were selected by a prescribed process for use in comparing nutrients and costs under the current Nutrition Standards and Meal Requirements with those under the recommended Meal Requirements.

School Breakfast Program The program under which participating schools operate a nonprofit breakfast program in accordance with 7 CFR Part 220.

School Food Authority The governing body that is responsible for the administration of one or more schools and that has the legal authority to operate the school meal programs therein or that is otherwise approved by the Food and Nutrition Service of the U.S. Department of Agriculture to operate the school meal programs.

School Meals Initiative The School Meals Initiative includes the current regulations that define how the *Dietary Guidelines for Americans* and other Nutrition Standards apply to school meals. This initiative includes actions that support state agencies, school food authorities, and communities in improving school meals and encouraging children to improve their overall diets.

School Meals-Target Mean Intake Statistically derived target 24-hour intakes for nutrients that were used in developing the Nutrient Targets for school meals.

Schoolchildren Children in the United States who are school age (typically 5–18 years old).

Side Dish(es) Currently, any menu item (except condiments) that is offered in addition to the entrée and fluid milk under the nutrient-based menu planning approaches for the school lunch or any menu item offered in addition to fluid milk for the school breakfast.

State Agency State agency refers to (1) the state educational agency or (2) any other agency of the state that has been designated by the governor or other appropriate executive or legislative authority of the state and approved by the U.S. Department of Agriculture to administer the program in schools.

Target Median Intake Statistically derived target intake for nutrients used to plan diets for groups.

Tolerable Upper Intake Level The highest daily nutrient intake level that is likely to pose no risk of adverse health effects to almost all individuals in the general population.

Traditional Food-Based Menu Planning Approach One of the two current food-based menu planning approaches established by the U.S. Department of Agriculture that use meal patterns with food items from specific food components in quantities appropriate for established age-grade groups.

Usual Nutrient Intake Data based on 24-hour recall and statistically adjusted to better estimate usual intake; for this report, reference to nutrient intake includes energy (calories).

Appendix B

Biographical Sketches of Committee Members

VIRGINIA A. STALLINGS, M.D., is the Jean A. Cortner Endowed Chair in Pediatric Gastroenterology, Director of the Nutrition Center at the Children's Hospital of Philadelphia, and Director of the Office of Faculty Development at the Children's Hospital of Philadelphia Research Institute. Dr. Stallings is also a Professor of Pediatrics at the University of Pennsylvania School of Medicine. Her research interests include pediatric nutrition, evaluation of dietary intake and energy expenditure, and nutrition-related chronic disease. Her current research is funded by the National Institutes of Health (NIH) and foundations. Dr. Stallings served on numerous Institute of Medicine (IOM) projects including the Committee on Nutrition Services for Medicare Beneficiaries (chair), the Committee on the Scientific Basis for Dietary Risk Eligibility Criteria for WIC Programs (chair), the Committee to Review the WIC Food Packages (member), Nutrition Standards for Foods in Schools (chair), and the Food and Nutrition Board. Dr. Stallings earned a B.S. in nutrition and foods from Auburn University, an M.S. in human nutrition and biochemistry from Cornell University, and an M.D. from the School of Medicine of the University of Alabama in Birmingham. She completed a pediatric residency at the University of Virginia and a pediatric nutrition fellowship at the Hospital for Sick Children, Toronto, Ontario. Dr. Stallings is board certified in pediatrics and clinical nutrition. She is an IOM member and recently received the Foman Nutrition Award from the American Academy of Pediatrics.

KAREN WEBER CULLEN, Dr.P.H., R.D., is Associate Professor of pediatrics at the Children's Nutrition Research Center, Baylor College of

Medicine. Her primary research interest area is the prevention of obesity and diet-related chronic diseases. Current projects include the exploration of strategies to increase school breakfast consumption in middle schools; the development and evaluation of a website on healthy eating and physical activity for high school students; the evaluation of a web-based program on healthy eating for African American families; and dissemination of a video intervention on improving the family home food environment and food parenting tips for Cooperative Extension Expanded Food and Nutrition Education Program classes. Dr. Cullen's professional memberships include the Society for Nutrition Education, the Society for Behavioral Medicine, the American Dietetic Association, and the Texas Dietetic Association (Distinguished Scientist Award in 2001). She serves as a member of the Dannon Institute Scientific Council, the Dannon Institute Schools Committee, and the Schools Committee of the Alliance for a Healthier Generation. Dr. Cullen has an M.S. in nutrition from Case Western Reserve University and a Dr.P.H. in health promotion and health education from The University of Texas School of Public Health.

ROSEMARY DEDERICHS, B.A., is Director of the Food Services Department for the Minneapolis Public School District, Minnesota. She has worked with the school district for 24 years, serving as a food service assistant, site manager, multisite coordinator, and operations manager. Ms. Dederichs began her career in schools as a certified elementary school teacher. At present she is certified as a State and City Food Manager and certified at Level III in Child Nutrition through the National School Nutrition Association. Ms. Dederichs is a former executive board member of the Minnesota School Nutrition Association and serves on the Gold Star Advisory Board for General Mills, Inc. She received the Golden Apple Award for Nutrition Education from the Minnesota School Nutrition Association and a Community Partner Star Award from the University of Minnesota School of Public Health, Environmental Health Sciences Division, in recognition of her contributions to the guidance of Minneapolis Public Schools students. She was also a corecipient of the Allina Health Systems 2006 Healthy Community Award for developing healthier menus for her students. She was a member of the IOM Committee on Nutrition Standards for Foods in Schools. Ms. Dederichs has a B.A. in psychology from Mundelein College of Loyola University and conducted additional studies in education at Northern Illinois University, College of DuPage, and Elmhurst College.

MARY KAY FOX, M.Ed., is Senior Researcher at Mathematica Policy Research Inc. Ms. Fox has more than 20 years of research experience with child nutrition and school programs and is a recognized authority on the USDA school meal programs. She directed the second School Nutrition

Dietary Assessment Study (SNDA-II), was co-principal investigator of the recently completed third SNDA study (SNDA-III), and is currently directing the fourth SNDA study (SNDA-IV). She has conducted research on the adequacy and quality of diets consumed by school-aged children and the contribution of school meals and competitive foods consumed at school to children's dietary intakes and obesity risk. Her nutrition expertise extends to preschool-aged children, infants, and toddlers. She led nutrition substudies on two comprehensive national studies of the Child and Adult Care Feeding Program and serves as a co-principal investigator on the 2008 Feeding Infants and Toddler Study. Awards include a distinguished service award from the American Dietetic Association and Recognized Young Dietitian of the Year from the Massachusetts Dietetic Association. Ms. Fox has a B.S. in nutrition and dietetics from Mundelein College of Loyola University and an M.Ed. in nutrition from Tufts University.

LISA HARNACK, Dr.P.H., R.D., M.P.H., is Associate Professor and Director of the Nutrition Coordinating Center, Department of Epidemiology and Community Health, University of Minnesota, Minneapolis. Dr. Harnack's primary research interests focus on assessment and evaluation of dietary behaviors and dietary intake, particularly as they relate to prevention of chronic disease and obesity. Dr. Harnack is a member of the American Dietetic Association, the American Society for Nutrition, and the Association of Faculties of Graduate Programs in Public Health Nutrition. She has M.P.H. and Dr.P.H. degrees in public health nutrition from the University of California at Berkeley. She is a registered dietitian.

GAIL G. HARRISON, Ph.D., is Professor in the Department of Community Health Sciences at the UCLA School of Public Health and Senior Research Scientist at the UCLA Center for Health and Policy Research. She is Director of UCLA's Center for Global and Immigrant Health. Previously, she was professor in the Department of Family and Community Medicine at the University of Arizona. Dr. Harrison has worked extensively in the area of dietary and nutritional assessment of diverse populations. Dr. Harrison is a former member of the Food and Nutrition Board and has served on several of its committees, including the Committee on International Nutrition Programs, the Committee to Review the Risk Criteria for the WIC Program, the Committee on Implications of Dioxin in the Food Supply, and the Committee to Revise the WIC Food Packages. She has served in various advisory capacities for NIH and the U.S. Department of Agriculture (USDA), consulted with the World Health Organization and UNICEF, and has worked in Egypt, the Sudan, Iran, Indonesia, and Lesotho in addition to the United States. Dr. Harrison has an M.N.S. (nutritional sciences) from Cornell University and a Ph.D. in physical anthropology from the University of Arizona. She also serves on the Board of the California Food Policy Advocates organization. Dr. Harrison is a Fellow of the American Society for Nutrition and an IOM Member.

MARY ARLINDA HILL, M.S., S.N.S., is Executive Director of child nutrition services for Jackson Public Schools (Jackson, Mississippi). She has held this position for 26 years. Prior to beginning a career in school nutrition in 1983, she taught commercial food courses to vocational and technical students. Ms. Hill has been an active member of the Mississippi School Nutrition Association, serving as their president in 1988–1989, and is past president of the National School Nutrition Association, serving a term from July 2007 to July 2008. She is currently serving as President of the School Nutrition Foundation from August 2008 to July 2009. Ms. Hill has a B.S. and M.S. in home economics from the University of Southern Mississippi and is credentialed as a School Nutrition Specialist (S.N.S.). She also teaches recertification courses for food service managers at Hinds Community College in Jackson, Mississippi, and at Holmes Community College in Ridgeland, Mississippi. She has also served on numerous task forces and committees for the Office of Child Nutrition, State Department of Education for Mississippi, on related child nutrition issues. Ms. Hill is also very active in her community, with membership in various organizations, and serves on several boards of directors for nonprofit organizations.

HELEN H. JENSEN, Ph.D., is Professor in the Department of Economics, College of Agriculture and Life Sciences, at Iowa State University (ISU). Dr. Jensen is also head of the Food and Nutrition Policy Division in the Center for Agricultural and Rural Development at ISU. Dr. Jensen's research concerns food demand and consumption, food assistance and nutrition policies, food security, and the economics of food safety and hazard control. She is a member of the Board of Directors of the American Agricultural Economics Association, and serves on the editorial board of a number of professional journals. Dr. Jensen has been a member of the National Research Council's (NRC's) Committee on National Statistics' panel to review USDA's measurement of food insecurity and hunger, other NRC committees related to the U.S. sheep industry, animal health and diseases, and the executive board of the American Council on Consumer Interests. She is currently a member of NRC's Committee on Ranking FDA Product Categories Based on Health Consequences, and recently served on the IOM Committee to Review the WIC Food Packages. Dr. Jensen holds a B.A. in economics from Carleton College, an M.S. in agricultural and applied economics from the University of Minnesota, and a Ph.D. in agricultural economics from the University of Wisconsin-Madison.

RONALD E. KLEINMAN, M.D., is Physician in Chief of the Massachusetts General Hospital for Children, Chair of the Department of Pediatrics and Chief of the Pediatric Gastroenterology and Nutrition Unit at Massachusetts General Hospital, and the Charles Wilder Professor of Pediatrics at Harvard Medical School. His major areas of research interest include gastrointestinal immunology, nutritional support of infants and children, and nutrition and public health policy. Dr. Kleinman's professional affiliations include the American Gastroenterological Association, the American Association for the Study of Liver Diseases, the North American Society for Pediatrics Gastroenterology and Nutrition, the Society for Pediatric Research, and the American Pediatric Society. He is the author of more than 150 peer-reviewed publications, chapters, monographs, and textbooks. He has been a member of the Medical Advisory Group on Diet and Nutrition Guidelines in Cancer for the American Cancer Society, National Cholesterol Advisory Committee, and a member of the Board of Trustees for the Global Child Nutrition Foundation and Project Bread. Dr. Kleinman served as Chair of the Committee on Nutrition for the American Academy of Pediatrics and is the editor of the fourth, fifth, and sixth editions of the Academy's *Pediatric Nutrition Handbook*. He consults for the Grain Food Foundation, Sesame Street Foundation, Beech Nut, the Burger King External Advisory Board, and General Mills. A graduate of Trinity College in Hartford, Connecticut, Dr. Kleinman earned his M.D. from New York Medical College and completed his residency and chief residency in pediatrics at the Albert Einstein College of Medicine in New York and his fellowship in Pediatric Gastroenterology and Nutrition at the Massachusetts General Hospital, Harvard Medical School, Boston, Massachusetts.

GEORGE P. McCABE, Ph.D., is Professor of Statistics, Department of Statistics, and Associate Dean for Academic Affairs for the College of Science at Purdue University. Current research interests include applications of statistics in a variety of areas with particular emphasis on nutrition. He is a fellow of the American Statistical Association and a member of the Institute of Mathematical Statistics, the American Society for Quality, the New York Academy of Sciences, and the American Association for the Advancement of Science. He is the coauthor of a widely used introductory statistical text and more than 150 publications, ranging from statistical theory to a meta-analysis comparing daily and weekly iron supplementation. He served on the IOM Committee on the Use of Dietary Reference Intakes in Nutrition Labeling. He has a Ph.D. in mathematical statistics from Columbia University.

SUZANNE P. MURPHY, Ph.D., R.D., is a Researcher and Professor at the Cancer Research Center of Hawaii at the University of Hawaii and director of the Nutrition Support Shared Resource at the center. Dr. Murphy's research interests include dietary assessment methodology, development of food and supplement composition databases, and nutritional epidemiology of chronic diseases (with emphasis on cancer and obesity). Dr. Murphy has served as a member of the National Nutrition Monitoring Advisory Council and the year 2000 Dietary Guidelines Advisory Committee. Currently she serves on the editorial board for *Nutrition Today* and is a contributing editor for *Nutrition Reviews*. She is a member of various professional organizations including the American Dietetic Association, the American Society for Nutrition, the American Public Health Association, the Society for Nutrition Education, and the Society for Epidemiological Research. Dr. Murphy has served on several IOM panels including the Subcommittee on Interpretation and Uses of Dietary Reference Intakes (as chair then member), the Subcommittee on Upper Safe Reference Levels of Nutrients (as member), and the Panel on Calcium and Related Nutrients (as member). She chaired the Committee to Review the WIC Food Packages and is a member of the Food and Nutrition Board. Dr. Murphy earned an M.S. in molecular biology from San Francisco State University and a Ph.D. in nutrition from the University of California at Berkeley. She is a registered dietitian.

ANGELA M. ODOMS-YOUNG, Ph.D., is an Assistant Professor in the Department of Kinesiology and Nutrition at the University of Illinois at Chicago. Prior to her current position, she was an Assistant Professor of Public Health and Health Education in the School of Nursing and Health Studies at Northern Illinois University (Dekalb, Illinois). Previously, Dr. Odoms-Young completed a Family Research Consortium Postdoctoral Fellowship focused on understanding family processes in diverse populations at the Pennsylvania State University and University of Illinois–Urbana-Champaign and a Community Health Scholars Fellowship in community-based participatory research at the University of Michigan School of Public Health. Her current research is focused on social, cultural, and environmental determinants of dietary practices and overweight/obesity in African American adults and children. She has extensive experience in conducting ethnographic and community-based research with low-income and minority populations. Dr. Odoms-Young is currently involved in several studies that examine the relationship between neighborhood/school food environments, individual dietary intake, and/or weight status. She received her M.S. and Ph.D. degrees from Cornell University in human nutrition and community nutrition, respectively.

YEONHWA PARK, Ph.D., is Assistant Professor and holds the F.J. Francis Endowed Chair in the Department of Food Sciences, University of Massachusetts, Amherst. Earlier she was assistant scientist in the Department of Biochemistry and then in the Food Research Institute at the University of Wisconsin-Madison. Her research interests have included conjugated linoleic acid for which she is a co-inventor on four patents (with license assigned to the Wisconsin Alumni Research Foundation). She is a member of the American Chemical Society, the American Oil Chemists Society (2003 Young Scientist Research Award), the Institute of Food Technologists, the American Heart Association, and the American Society for Nutrition and received the ILSI North America 2007 Future Leader Award. Dr. Park has an M.S. in pharmacy from Seoul National University and a Ph.D. in food sciences from the University of Wisconsin-Madison.

MARY JO TUCKWELL, M.P.H., R.D., previously served 18 years as Director of Food and Nutrition for the Eau Claire Area School District in Wisconsin; she is now a Senior Consultant for inTEAM Associates, Inc., a performance consulting group focusing on nutrition and management training in school food service. She also has experience in clinical dietetics and in academia, most recently as an adjunct professor and a dietetics internship preceptor at the University of Wisconsin-Stout. Recent professional activities included service on the Governor's Council on Physical Fitness and Health (Wisconsin) from 2003 to 2009 and on the Eau Claire City/County Board of Health (including vice president 1999–2008) from 1993 to 2008. She has been active in a number of professional associations including the American Dietetic Association, School Nutrition Association, and Society for Nutrition Education. She has a B.S. in dietetics from the University of Wisconsin-Stout and an M.P.H. from the University of California at Berkeley. She is a registered dietitian.

Appendixes C through Q are not printed in this book, but can be found on the CD at the back of the book or online at http://www.nap.edu.